W9-BHI-813

DON'T
DIET

DON'T DIET

DALE M. ATRENS, PH.D.

With an Introduction by
PETER VALK, M.D.

WILLIAM MORROW AND COMPANY, INC.
NEW YORK

Library of Congress Cataloging-in-Publication Data

Atrens, Dale M. (Dale Michael), 1941–
Don't diet.

Includes index.
1. Obesity. 2. Obesity—Psychological aspects.
3. Obesity—Social aspects. 4. Reducing. 5. Reducing diets. I. Title.
RC628.A87 1988 613.2'5 87-28220
ISBN 0-688-07469-3

Printed in the United States of America

2 3 4 5 6 7 8 9 10

BOOK DESIGN BY MARIE-HÉLÈNE FREDRICKS

CONTENTS

CHAPTER 2

CHAPTER 3

CHAPTER 4

CHAPTER 5

CHAPTER 6

CHAPTER 7

CHAPTER 8

INTRODUCTION

Fat has become a very negative word in our culture. The Western preference for slimness has grown to the point where bodily fat is seen as a weakness and even a vice. The "badness" of fat goes a long way: Fat means ugly, sexless, unhealthy, and weak. At its height, the anti-fat crusade takes on a religious tone: We are tainted by the presence of fat and hence we must mortify the flesh. Dieting is the only way to salvation. Unfortunately, for most people dieting doesn't work, so the person defined as fat—and that definition includes many people at some point in their lives—is left with no way out.

Dr. Atrens's book takes a fresh look at this gloom and doom. Dr. Atrens presents important data that have not reached the ears of the general public before and discusses basic findings that previously have often been misinterpreted. He starts with the basic nature of fat and its role in our bodies and proceeds through an analysis of what is means to be fat in our society. Along the way, he tackles most of the major frauds that have been foisted on us by the diet industry and takes a long look at how and why the diet gurus are thriving.

One of the most provocative aspects of this book is Dr. Atrens's critical examination of the relationship between fatness and health. He presents a great deal of information that is not easily accessible to the general reader and makes sense of confusing and often conflicting scientific data. His analysis leads to an understanding of fat and health in terms that have meaning for us. There is no doubt that fatness is best avoided. Extreme obesity is a serious disease in itself. Even less-severe obesity increases our chances of developing high blood pressure, high blood cholesterol, and diabetes, which in turn increase the risk of coronary heart disease. Unfortunately, most fat people can neither prevent nor reverse their fatness: Most fatness is probably metabolically determined and resists the onslaught of reduced food intake. Besides, few of us are equipped for daily, lifelong self-denial. As a result, many people cannot achieve significant and lasting weight loss by dieting, no matter how much they may want to, or even need to.

So, are fat people condemned to an unhealthy life and an early demise? Dr. Atrens's answer is a definite no. First, being fat does not necessarily mean being unhealthy. Second, fat people are not helpless just because the therapy of weight loss through dieting is not available to them. Dr. Atrens presents some important advice that applies to all people, fat or thin. Low intake of saturated fats and higher intake of complex carbohydrates, along with regular exercise, can do much to reduce the risk factors for heart disease, even without weight loss. Keeping track of blood pressure, blood sugar, and cholesterol should alert one to trouble brewing. Available evidence does not indicate that fatness itself causes atherosclerosis; neither does it suggest that the person who is otherwise well and has a healthy life-style is predisposed to heart disease because of obesity. However, overweight people are subjected to such a constant stream of anti-fat propaganda that they often give up hope of living a healthy life and therefore stop trying. This book should bring fat people back into the fold and increase our understanding of the care and feeding of our bodies.

This book spells out in detail the high emotional price of our society's approach to fatness. In our insistence on slimness, health has become confused with cosmetic motivations. We have set extremely demanding goals for ourselves, ones that are often unattainable, and we punish ourselves severely when we do not reach them. The misery and guilt created by the fear of fat are most obvious in the eating disorders anorexia nervosa and bulimia. These disorders are now epidemic among young women. There is little doubt that for each case of eating disorder, there are hundreds of other people who suffer quiet, chronic unhappiness. Overweight men and women are told to diet and lose weight, a goal that is beyond most normal, healthy people, and then have to face the cost of their failure: They are not just fat, but weak as well. They're ugly and unhealthy and they deserve it. This is a heavy burden to carry through life, in addition to all the other demands we make on ourselves. For millions of us, this amounts to a chronic attack on our self-esteem. Low self-esteem is a precursor of depression, which surely is even worse for you than weighing "too much." No one benefits from all these pressures, and Dr. Atrens helps us to start feeling better about our bodies, even if they are not "ideal." He shows us that to fail at dieting is the norm: It merely reflects how difficult it is to defeat our own physiology. Certainly those who fail should not be regarded as inadequate.

Dale Atrens is well qualified to write about fatness and fat people. His views have grown from twenty years' study of behavior and metabolism. He originally trained in psychology and obtained a Ph.D. for his work on brain-behavior relationships. Thereafter, his work continued to develop in the direction of psychobiology—the study of psychology and biology together. The major part of his career has involved the study of caloric intake and metabolism, and his interest in weight control is longstanding. He is an established and widely published researcher. In recognition of his outstanding achievements, Dr. Atrens was appointed reader in the department of psychology at the University of Sydney. There he heads an active interdisciplinary research group, investigating the psychobiology of energy balance. Besides his many contributions to scientific literature, he is the author of a recent textbook in neuroscience and another in psychology and he has lectured on these topics around the world. In many ways, this book is a return to his beginnings: the application of what he has learned to the way we see ourselves and each other.

You do not have to identify with every step in Dr. Atrens's arguments to gain from his conclusions. Fatness has become a big problem in Western society and, for many, our attitude toward it has become a bigger problem still. This book will remedy some of that.

—PETER VALK, M.D.

DON'T DIET

CHAPTER 1

WHY BE FAT?

In a world inundated by diet books one may reasonably question the need for yet another. By now the community at large should have a healthy skepticism for new wonder diets and all of their trappings. But it hasn't. Hope springs eternal, and each new book offers the same old promises of new secrets of beauty and health. There are millions of potential converts eagerly awaiting the newest diet messiah.

The international religious community of dieters is bound together by an uncommonly small creed: *Fat is evil. Slenderness is salvation.* The diet messiahs paint apocalyptic visions of doom visited upon those who refuse to purge themselves of the sin of fat. They paint visions of fulfillment and of the full bounty of social largesse visited upon those who choose to be saved. Beauty, love, and longevity are all there, simply awaiting your embrace.

The diet messiahs differ mainly in their prescription for the road to salvation. Some offer easy salvation without the hardship of diets and exercise. Others exact penance with rigorous dietary privation and assaultive exercise. The relative popularity of the easy routes versus the hard ones waxes and wanes in some sort of loose synchronization with political and economic cycles.

In spite of their superficial differences, the diet messiahs have one overriding similarity. They are united in their failure to arrest the spread of fat. Quite simply, if any of their prescriptions fulfilled their promises, we would all be saved. But they don't, and we aren't. Fat people should be an endangered species. Instead, they appear to be the wave of the future. Over the last thirty years, spectacular increases in the income of the diet industry have been accompanied by steady increases in the fatness of the population.

The purpose of this book is to foster some sane thinking in this insane area. Many of the assumptions underlying the international obsession with fat are both wrong and dangerous. Fat, in most cases, is not a health hazard, and weight loss is not a generally desirable ideal. The assumptions that fat is due to gluttony and sloth are without foundation. The view that all fat is ugly is an unnatural and unhealthy prejudice. Nor is it simply a matter of choosing to be fat or thin. Fatness and thinness are reflections of fundamental physiological processes over which we have surprisingly little control. Dieting and exercise have remarkably small and short-term effects on body weight. New research reveals that our ignorance about where fat comes from, its significance, and what to do about it has produced one of the most widespread, yet totally avoidable, sources of misery in our times.

The *psychobiological* approach of this book stresses the concurrent investigation of psychological and physiological factors. Such an approach should help to remove this subject from the morass of quackery in which it is now embedded. Hopefully, this will lead to a radical restructuring of how we view fatness and dieting. Herein lies the freedom from the tyranny of fat.

Fat Is Your Friend: The Physiology of Energy Storage

It may come as a surprise that fat exists for any other reason than to harass us. Fat is commonly viewed as a cross we bear, perhaps as a penalty for the misdeeds of our species. Fat is commonly portrayed as the physiological equivalent of original sin. In order to come to terms with our fat, it is first necessary to understand just what it is and what purpose it serves.

Like all animals, we continuously use energy, which we obtain from food. However, we eat only occasionally, and we must have a way of storing energy for use between meals. If we couldn't store energy, we would have to spend all our time eating. Take the tree shrew, for example. The tree shrew can store so little energy that, if it doesn't eat, it will starve to death in only a few hours. This means that tree shrews must spend virtually all their waking hours either eating or searching for food. This may be why tree shrews have produced so little great art or music.

Fortunately, humans store large amounts of energy, in the form of carbohydrates, fats, and protein. Our energy stores give us a degree of independence from food, which allows us to exploit our other abilities. Unlike the tree shrew, we can eat infrequently and we can also eat for fun. Our lives should be enhanced, not dominated by food. Alas, the current madness concerning eating, dieting, and fatness has made many of us more dominated by food than the tree shrew.

The central carbohydrate in energy metabolism is glucose. Glucose is mostly obtained through the digestion of sugars and starches, and is distributed by the bloodstream to every cell in our body. The cells use glucose for their immediate energy needs, and any excess is stored in the muscles and liver in an inactive form called *glycogen,* or in adipose tissue as fat. On demand, glycogen is converted back into glucose. However, our glycogen reserves are quite small. Consequently, they are only a short-term source of energy. A typical adult has about one pound of glycogen, which contains enough energy for twenty-four to forty-eight hours. The fact that humans can usually endure weeks of starvation indicates that we must have another, far larger energy store. This main energy storage is found in fat.

A typical 150-pound adult carries about twenty to forty pounds of fat. Although there are several different kinds of fat, our concern is with the *triglycerides*. Triglycerides are combinations of fatty acids and glycerol and are stored in adipose tissue.

Within the adipose tissue triglycerides are split and liberated fatty acids are stored in droplets within the fat cell. The size of the fat-cell droplets, and consequently the size of the fat cells themselves, varies widely depending on the level of their stores of fatty acids. On demand, the fatty acids supply energy to the body by entering into the same biochemical cycle as glucose.

Ultimately, fat and glucose are fully interchangeable as sources of energy. Excess glucose is stored as fat, and when energy is needed, fat can substitute for glucose. There is, however, one major exception to this general interchangeability. The brain is the only organ in the body that cannot use fatty acids for energy. The brain runs exclusively on glucose. This exception becomes very important when we consider the effects of dieting and starvation on brain function. These superficially simple energy-storage and retrieval processes are, in fact, enormously complex. They are regulated by an orchestra of nervous and hormonal processes.

Perhaps the most important characteristic of fat is that it is by far the most efficient form of energy storage. This results from the fact that fat is almost water-free. Water is, in a sense, dead weight because it has no energy value. In contrast, the other main energy-storage form, glycogen, is about 70 to 80 percent water. If all the energy in our fat were instead stored as glycogen, we would weigh nearly twice as much as we do now! Obviously, then, fat is an important evolutionary development. It helps us keep our weight down!

We have still another form of energy storage—protein. About 25 percent of our total energy reserves are in the form of protein. However, unlike glycogen and fat, protein is not a useful everyday energy-storage form. Protein is mainly stored as muscle and using protein for energy would inevitably destroy muscle. Since muscle is working weight, its destruction impairs a wide range of functions. Prolonged muscle destruction ultimately produces death. Using your own protein for energy is a bit like being at sea and using your boat for firewood. On the other hand, using glycogen and fat for energy actually increases physiological efficiency by reducing ballast in the form of nonworking weight.

Sparing your own protein during starvation makes good sense. However, the "wisdom of the body" can sometimes be defeated. In diets, particularly severe ones, significant amounts of muscle may be sacrificed long before fat stores are exhausted. This failure to spare the protein stored in muscles may be partly responsible for the unusual fatigue and lethargy often produced by radical diets. This will be discussed at length in chapter 5.

The foregoing considerations show that fat is our friend because it is a lightweight, highly efficient form of energy storage.

Fat is also our friend for other reasons. First, by smoothing out the stark irregularities of our skeleton, fat serves a cosmetic function. Fat also has a mechanical advantage, since it protects our vulnerable joints. Additionally, fat is good thermal insulation. Fat deposits just below the skin minimize heat loss in the cold. So, fat is good for us in many ways. It is time we stopped thinking of it as an adversary.

By this time you should be feeling a little better about your fat. Evolution wouldn't have given you a bad body. But evolution does act in ways that are considerably slower than the vagaries of fashion. When fashion and physiology become out of synch, trouble begins.

Slenderness as an ideal has waxed and waned in the fashion industry for centuries. The latest broad cycle of this aesthetic roller coaster began in the 1920s, whereas the evolution of the human body began some millions of years earlier. Consequently, it should come as no great surprise that our bodies do not always live up to the demands of late-twentieth-century fashion. For the great majority of human history, the aesthetics of body fat have had to take second place to the struggle for survival. It is only in very recent times that we have been able to afford the luxury of trying to vary our body weight and fat stores in order to meet aesthetic, rather than survival, needs (see chapter 8).

It is clear that, in affluent societies at least, it is no longer necessary to be able to endure four to five weeks of starvation. Yet, given a typical body-fat content of 20 to 30 percent, that is about how long most of us would last. Imagine us, instead, as having a body-fat content of 2 to 3 percent. We could still safely endure several days' starvation—much more than any of us is ever likely to experience. However, a body-fat content of 2 to 3 percent, while safe according to the above criteria, would make you look so emaciated that you would be considered strange anywhere but in the world of women's fashions. Any man with this little fat would likely be hospitalized. Yet Zulu hunters are built rather like this. They carry just enough fat to see them through a long gazelle chase. Any more would slow them down and any less would leave them with inadequate range.

Zulus have a clear aesthetic head start on the rest of us if, in the quest for beauty, our value system demands extreme slenderness. This demand is particularly imperative for women. We do not have the body composition of Zulus, nor can we acquire it. That is the source of our woes. If we can hang on for another ten to twenty thousand years, our bodies might make the transition from fat to lean. But, for the moment, don't hold your breath. In that light I like to think of this book as my contribution to helping us cope with the strains of the next ten to twenty thousand years.

How Fat Should You Be? Defining and Measuring Fatness

This is a deceptively difficult question. It's so difficult that I can't really answer it, and neither can anyone else. A lot of people, however, claim to have the answer. If you fit their definition of having enough fat, you are entitled to be smug. If you have too much fat, you are expected to be ashamed or frightened. Fat people are told that their fatness indicates that there is something wrong with them. They are expected to remedy their deficiency and maintain a normal or ideal weight.

There is a simple way around the shame and fear generated by failing to comply with the prevailing definition of an ideal weight: Find another definition of an ideal weight that you find more congenial. It's not all that hard to do, since ideal weights are essentially just arbitrary anyhow. The simple fact is that while we all may have an ideal weight, it is so highly individual that it is not to be obtained from any tables. In a species as heterogeneous as ours, there are likely to be millions of ideal weights. The most comprehensive tables have maybe a few hundred ideal weights, which means that they are probably valid for only a tiny fraction of the general population.

The very fact that so many people regard ideal-weight tables with virtual reverence is evidence enough of the absurdity that abounds in this area. Like any area in which there is enough fear and ignorance, fat has become a lucrative hunting ground for quacks and charlatans. Fat quackery is, unfortunately, not just an idle form of mischief. It feeds upon and creates untold misery. Millions of people are tormented by absurd and dangerous expectations of what their bodies can and should be like.

The ideal-weight tables that terrorize the community consist of a range of weights for various ages and heights. There are, of course, separate tables for men and women. These data are derived from insurance company records. Ultimately, these records attempt to relate body weight to the profitability of insuring someone. This is the only sense in which the weights presented in these tables are ideal. They have financial utility. Insurance companies use the tables much the way a gambler uses a racing form. Since they are gambling on your life, they are particularly interested in anything that will improve their chances of winning.

The weight-for-age tables may well have helped the insurance companies to be winners. However, these tables have been badly misinterpreted. They say almost nothing about whether fat is a health hazard. They merely say that of those people who take out life insurance, the heavier ones are poorer risks. To say that this is an effect of excess fat or that these data apply to the population as a whole is not justified. This most important message continues to go ignored by many health professionals and almost all of the general public. It is not at all a trivial or academic issue, but rather is one of the two main reasons why so many people are engaged in hand-to-hand combat with their fat (see chapter 2).

Perhaps because the insurance companies have been so financially successful, the validity of their ideal-weight tables is rarely questioned. Or at least the questioning of these tables is largely confined to narrow academic circles. We will examine the validity of statistical definitions of overweight. Do they really tell us anything meaningful?

One problem with statistical, or normative, definitions of overweight (that is, those used by insurance companies) is that they are, at best, applicable to those people who apply for life insurance. This group is not at all representative of the population as a whole (see Chapter 2). Generalizing from such a highly selected group about the population at large can lead to serious errors. In addition, these definitions are entirely retrospective, so they inevitably lag far behind a rapidly changing population.

Recently in the United States, for example, the desirable weights in the life insurance tables were revised sharply upward for both men and women. By one stroke of an actuarial pen, the health status of the entire American people appeared to improve dramatically and instantaneously! Millions of people were suddenly pronounced risk-free and healthy, whereas the night before, these same people were considered to be endangered and unhealthy! This would appear to be easily the most rapid evolutionary development in the history of our species. Either that or it was a major miracle. Yet, at this extraordinary announcement, the public shrugged a sigh of relief rather than a more appropriate guffaw of disbelief. The credulity of the general public with respect to fatness is difficult to overestimate.

The revered weight-for-age tables suffer from other serious deficiencies as well. For example, how do you take into account the effects of different heights and frame sizes? To correct the data for the effects of these obvious variables would make the tables extremely large and unwieldy. They would have to be at least three-dimensional. To correctly determine whether people are over or under their "ideal" weight, you would also have to know their ideal height and frame size (see below). To suggest that someone has an ideal height or frame size is absurd. It may be no less absurd to suggest that they have an ideal weight.

One way of avoiding the dizzying difficulties of complex, multidimensional tables is to reduce all the data to a single number, such as the *ponderal index*. The ponderal index, which is also sometimes known, after its inventor, as *Quetelet's index,* is obtained by dividing weight (in kilograms) by the square of height (in meters). This most convenient figure (W/H^2) is based on two easily obtained measurements—height and weight. Anyone who can multiply and divide can calculate ponderal indices. The first question that should be asked of this index is how well does it correlate with other indices of fatness? The answer is, not very well.

The inadequacy of the ponderal index as a measure of fatness should not be surprising in light of its origins. Although the expression W/H^2 is mathematically precise, it is conceptually flimsy. The use of H^2 comes from the fact that simply dividing by H appeared to make tall people more likely to be fat. On the other hand, dividing by H^3 appeared to make short people more likely to be fat. In other words, any validity the ponderal index has is only after the fact. It was modified to fit the available data. These data have since changed, so the fit of the index to the data is now even poorer than it was originally. Such a cut-and-fit index is hardly the stuff of which great truths are made. The ponderal index is mainly useful in explaining truths that are derived from the ponderal index. Its scant validity is almost entirely circular.

These inadequacies are further compounded by the need to correct for frame size. It is reasonable that someone with a small frame should weigh less than someone with a large one. People are often described as being "big-boned" or "small-boned." It should then be easy to adjust ponderal indices for frame size. Alas, there is no generally accepted measure of frame size. In the rare cases where frame size is even considered, it is almost invariably based on an eyeball estimate; that is, it is usually little more than a guess.

The question recurs as to what are reasonable norms for human body weight? The answer is that there aren't any. It seems almost absurd that we do not really know an ideal weight for anyone. This, of course, means that notions such as overweight are not very meaningful. Overweight only makes sense in relation to normal or ideal weight but the problem is that we lack an adequate definition of what a normal or ideal weight is. There is no shortage of definitions. There is merely a shortage of *adequate* definitions. Indeed, the present analysis suggests that an adequate definition of *normal weight* is unlikely ever to be made. Sometime in the future it may be possible to estimate what an individual's ideal weight is, but you can be sure that such an estimate will not be based on averages derived from insurance company records.

The folly that arbitrary measures of an ideal weight lead to is nicely reflected in the classic Build and Blood Pressure Study. This study turns out to be very important to the question of fat as a health hazard (see chapter 2). According to this study, when fatness was expressed as a percentage of ideal weight, tall people were seen as more likely to have high blood pressure. When fatness was expressed in terms of the ponderal index, short people were seen as more likely to have high blood pressure!

With any normative measure there is always the central question of what is normal and what is abnormal. That this is not a trivial question is illustrated by the following example.

Using 20 percent over "normal" weight as the criterion of overweight, the revered Metropolitan Life Insurance tables indicate that about 35 percent of adult Americans are too fat. Using the exact same criterion for the data of the Build and Blood Pressure Study shows that only about 10 percent are too fat! Depending on the source of the data, the incidence of overweight varies by more than threefold. This raises the question of whose data are right? In this case the answer is neither. Alternately, one could say that they were both right for their respective populations but that neither applies to the population as a whole. However, we are continually being told that either or both of these studies depicts general relationships that hold for everyone. Something is amiss. There is something fundamentally wrong with normative measures of fatness even when they are mathematically "adjusted." Even the most sophisticated mathematics cannot compensate for an inadequate initial concept such as "normal" weight. If there is no such thing as normal weight, then all the mathematizing in the world will not legitimate it.

Similarly, it is easy to determine the average height of any group of people, but to call this average a *normal* height implies that there is something wrong with those who are not *average*. That those whose height is not average are different from the average is, of course, indisputable. However, to suggest that there is something wrong with them is another thing altogether.

Being fat does not necessarily mean that there is something wrong with you, nor does it necessarily mean that you should try to get thin. In most cases, it just means that you are fat. On the other hand, there is a small minority of fat people who are clearly the victim of a pathological process. If your weight is 50 percent fat, you may be one of these genuinely afflicted few. The continuing confusion between the genuinely unfortunate, small minority and the simply fat, large majority works to the detriment of all of us. There is another, somewhat larger minority who can genuinely benefit from weight loss (see chapter 2). These minority groups could really improve their health by losing weight. However, most people who are desperately trying to lose weight have no legitimate reason to do so. Perhaps this is just as well, since as we shall see in chapters 5 through 7 weight loss is almost always an unattainable goal.

Another source of error in the normative measures is that they are measures of weight, not fatness. That weight and fatness are not the same should be fairly obvious. Athletes, for example, may have very high weights and ponderal indices, yet have little body fat. In contrast, elderly, sedentary people may have low weights and ponderal indices, yet be quite fat. It's really quite simple. If you want to talk about fatness, you should measure fat, not weight. The problem is that directly measuring fat is difficult. The only really precise way to measure it is to homogenize the whole body in a blender and then extract the fats from the rest using special solvents. Obviously, we must rely on indirect and less lethal procedures for such measuring.

Unfortunately, indirect measures of body fat are not very precise and can only be validated by occasional comparison with direct procedures. This is rarely done. Complete carcass analyses appear to have been done on only six human cadavers. As a result, our knowledge of human body composition and the validity of indirect measures of body fat is still at a primitive level. All of this means that our obsession with fat is based on remarkably frail foundations.

The simplest indirect measure of body fat is skinfold thickness. This measure is based on the assumption that most body fat is stored just beneath the skin, so that if you pinch a measured length of skin, the thickness of the fold should indicate the amount of fat underneath it. This technique is popular in that it only requires a pair of calipers and some practice. Further, skinfold thickness correlates better with other, more precise measures of body fat than do any of the statistical-normative measures described above.

In spite of these advantages, skinfold thickness remains a rather crude way of measuring body fat. Its precision varies considerably at different places on the body and in different groups. Even trained observers can come up with quite different measures on the same subjects. We find ourselves in the strange position where everyone is interested in fat, everyone thinks they are talking about it, but almost nobody really is.

There is one fairly low-tech, yet quite precise measure of body fat. It is called *densitometry*. This procedure is based on Archimedes' principle. All you need is a fairly large water tank and a healthy, cooperative subject. First, you determine total body volume by immersing the subject in water; then, when you divide volume into weight, you are given the weight per unit of volume or density.

The logic of interpreting body density is refreshingly straightforward. Since fat is relatively water-free and muscle is relatively water-laden, fat is less dense than muscle. Consequently, a fat body will be less dense than a muscular body. This is why fat people float better. Although densitometry requires rather special facilities and cannot be used on everyone, it nevertheless remains one of the most precise measures of fat available. Unfortunately, it is too rarely used. Expediency is usually the name of the game, although it often shows little respect for the truth.

There are also, on the horizon, several high-tech measures of body fat. Body imaging with nuclear techniques and ultrasound offer considerable promise of at last providing precise measures of what fat is all about. Until reasonably precise measures of body fat are more widely used, this area of study will remain riddled with fundamental uncertainty. Imagine studying temperature without a decent thermometer. This is the situation in the fat business.

Now that you are aware of the formidable difficulties in measuring body fat, as opposed to simple weight, it may be appropriate to tell you that this distinction probably doesn't matter very much. In most cases it is only extreme levels of fatness that should reasonably be considered a health hazard. This sort of fatness can be seen a city block away; it doesn't require sophisticated or precise measurement.

Fat as an aesthetic issue is something entirely different (see chapter 8) from fat as a health hazard. The main concepts pertaining to both these fundamental issues of fatness are in a remarkably primitive state. We are in the unfortunate situation of having a reasonably good technology that is at the mercy of a hopelessly inadequate set of concepts and values. Almost everyone wants less fat. Yet the nearly universal desire to lose weight is generated by twisted aesthetics and misinterpreted health data. This motivation is nearly as invalid as it is strong. However, in spite of all of this misplaced urgency, we don't know how to get there. There is no good way to lose weight. We are stampeding off in all directions, and a lot of people are getting hurt in the stampede. The concepts and values underlying fatophobia are in need of a drastic overhaul. That is what this book is all about.

WHO IS FAT? SOCIAL FACTORS THAT MAKE YOU FAT

Some people and some groups of people are far more likely to be fat than others. Fatness is not evenly distributed in any society. This is precisely why we are so bothered about it. If everyone weighed the same, regardless of whether it was a lot or a little, nobody would care. The striking differences in fatness between individuals and groups suggest some factors that may contribute to fatness. Some of these factors may be avoidable, others are not, but they are all instructive.

HEREDITY

It is a common observation that fatness runs in families. If neither of your parents is fat, you have about a 10 percent chance of becoming fat. If one of your parents is fat, you have about a 50 percent chance of becoming fat. With two fat parents, your liability is about 80 percent. In any case, you can't do anything about your genetic makeup. Although few professionals would dispute these basic findings, their interpretation is a matter of hot dispute.

That fatness runs in families may indicate a genetic contribution to fatness. It could also indicate that the same environment that made the parents fat will likely make the children fat. Parents and children generally share the same environment as well as the same genes. Fat pet owners tend to have fat pets, yet the owners and pets obviously have different genetic makeups. A more reasonable interpretation of these similarities is that there are common fat-promoting factors in the environment of owners and pets alike.

Once again we come to grips with the hoary old issue of nature versus nurture. In the case of fatness, the nature-nurture issue is of critical importance. For example, if people are fat because of a genetic predisposition, making them slim involves overcoming their genetic liability. Admitting a genetic influence on fatness leads to a distinct fatalism. This fatalism destroys the motivation to get slim. If anything is essential to slimming, it is unwavering motivation. If fatness does reflect a genetic bias, diets could only be seen as doomed to failure from the outset.

For the above reason, many professionals in the fat business are reluctant to acknowledge anything more than minor genetic effects on fatness. This rather curious head-in-the-sand approach is a bit like a high jumper refusing to accept the law of gravity because of its inconvenient implications. The facts ultimately stand by themselves, whether we like them or not. These facts are not absolutely unequivocal, but they certainly strongly suggest a major genetic contribution to fatness.

Numerous studies of twins point to a genetic contribution to both fatness and slenderness. Fraternal twins are much more likely to have similar weights than are nontwin siblings. Identical twins are even more likely to have similar weights. Clearly, increasing degrees of genetic similarity make for increasing similarity of body weight. In the case of twins, the effects of environment should be pretty much the same.

The genetic contribution to body weight (and presumably fatness) is even more impressive in the case of identical twins who have been separated at an early age. Even though the twins are reared in quite different environments, they still show very similar weights. In fact, the effects of separate rearing on the weights of identical twins is about the same as the effects of separate rearing on their height! These findings show how genetic effects can dominate over environmental ones.

When skinfold thickness (which is a better index of body fat) is used instead of weight, the genetic effect is even more impressive. The difference between skinfold thickness in pairs of identical twins is about one-third that of nonidentical twins. This points to an inescapable conclusion: Some people have a definite predisposition toward fatness. At a practical level, such a strong genetic tendency may well be very difficult to overcome. The failure of thousands of different weight-loss procedures attests to this difficulty.

The strength of a genetic tendency toward fatness can be seen in the nonfat brothers and sisters of fat children. Many of the nonfat children have the same highly efficient metabolism that contributes to the fatness of their fat siblings (see chapter 4). However, the nonfat children manage to disguise their genetic tendency by eating less. These children appear to be metabolically wired to be fat.

There is another rather curious and very important piece of information to emerge from the most recent genetic investigations. There are different types of fatness, and these various types have quite different genetic profiles. People are fat for a variety of reasons, so no simple or single explanation will apply to everyone. Consequently, the daily showers of pious pronouncements that fat is good, bad, or indifferent at best only apply to some fat people.

Many fat people are not uniformly fat. Some tend to have fat limbs, whereas others tend to have fat bodies. In males, body or trunk fat has a particularly strong genetic component. If you are a male with a father who has a fat body, you are more likely to inherit that than if your father had fat limbs. In females, limb fat appears to be more strongly inheritable. Interestingly, these genetic associations appear to strengthen with age. By their late teens, children of fat parents are three times more likely to be fat than are children of lean parents. By middle age, this threefold difference has increased to a sevenfold or eightfold difference. This is important, because it suggests that although the genetic influence may be temporarily suppressed, it eventually expresses itself.

EARLY EXPERIENCE

Just as you cannot control the genes that may predispose you to being fat, you also have no control over a variety of fat-predisposing events that occurred around the time of your birth. The very existence of these factors indicates that certain environmental events are important and that fatness is not totally genetically determined. The problem is that by the time most people are concerned about being fat, these critical events are long since past and they may well be irrevocable.

Mothers who were heavy before pregnancy are more likely to give birth to heavy infants. This fact is firmly embedded in folklore. Since fat infants are widely considered to be healthy, expectant mothers in many cultures are encouraged to gain weight. Even in mothers who are not heavy before pregnancy, a high rate of weight gain early in pregnancy increases the likelihood of the child being heavy. All of this suggests that the critical fat-predisposing events occur in the early stages of pregnancy.

One might well imagine that starvation early in pregnancy

would produce a permanent tendency toward being slender. Strangely, quite the opposite seems to occur. These data come from a fascinating study of 300,000 Dutch military recruits who were born during World War II. Their mothers had all experienced starvation at some time during pregnancy. Maternal starvation, particularly early in pregnancy, produces an apparently permanent tendency toward fatness in the child. Thus, either rapid maternal weight gain or starvation early in pregnancy predisposes the child to fatness. This raises the possibility that the critical signal that results in a fat child is not the mother's nutritional status per se but the presence of nutritional stress.

It is easy enough to see the adaptive value of a starved mother producing fat children. If the mother experienced starvation, it is quite likely that the child will too. In this case the fat child has a valuable head start. On the other hand, why a mother who gained weight rapidly in pregnancy would produce a fat child is not at all clear. If the mother is well fed, it is likely that the environment will support the child too. In this case being fat is of no particular advantage. This curiosity may indicate that the body cannot discriminate well between different types of stress. In response to nutritional stress, the body takes the safe way out by setting up the child to be fat. Fat is safe.

The implications of the above data for health are rather different from what we have generally been led to believe. Let us consider the health of fat infants. Here the popular wisdom turns out to be well founded. Fat infants are less likely to suffer from almost all postnatal problems. Their overall advantage is indicated by the fact that they have a lower mortality rate. Furthermore, there appears to only a weak relationship between infantile fatness and adult fatness. Most infants lose their baby fat, whereas fat adults typically acquire most of their fat later in life. In other words, a fat baby is a healthy baby and is not particularly likely to become a fat adult.

This is all very much at odds with contemporary behavior concerning maternal fat. The prevalent fear and loathing of fat is once again generating an unhealthy situation. A fat mother is commonly considered to be both ugly and unhealthy. The fat-blighted mother is also held in suspicion of willfully spreading her contagion to her child. We've already shown that this view has no basis in fact. In spite of its irrationality, however, this view led to a vogue of dieting during pregnancy. In the 1970s many pregnant women were coerced into rather severe diets. The object of the dieting was to produce skinny infants. This is in spite of the fact that skinny infants have a higher mortality rate. This madness is further compounded by the evidence that maternal starvation is, if anything, likely to produce children that develop into fat adults.

There is yet another, even uglier aspect of this poor logic. A dieting mother inevitably burns up her own fat when the diet has exhausted her carbohydrate reserves. Using fat for energy elevates blood ketones. High maternal ketone levels have been reported to have adverse effects on the intelligence of the child. The net result of the prevalent irrationality about fat during pregnancy is that we have created a health hazard. Such treatment-produced (iatrogenic) health hazards are the main harvest of the popular attitudes toward fat.

Even though fat children do not necessarily become fat adults, there is still a fairly widespread view that if adult fatness is due to overeating, this unfortunate habit must have been learned early in life. Consequently, there is considerable interest in the relation between infant feeding patterns and adult fatness.

There is a great deal of evidence to support the adage (mine) that says, "Spare the breast and spoil the child." Babies who are bottle-fed usually weigh considerably more than breast-fed babies. The reasons for this emphasize the importance of packaging: Unlike the breast, the bottle gives a clear indication as to whether it is empty. There is a common tendency to encourage the infant to finish the bottle, even though he or she may neither need nor want to. In contrast, the mother is more likely to discontinue breastfeeding when the infant shows signs of satiation. If left to their own devices, infants appear to regulate their energy intake quite well. However, infants probably have less ability than adults to compensate for overfeeding, and the bottle encourages overfeeding.

There is another, less obvious reason why bottle-feeding may predispose infants to fatness. Infant formulas are very imprecise imitations of breast milk. The proteins in human milk are unique and cannot be imitated by products formulated from cow's milk. In further contrast to formulas, the composition of breast milk varies over the day and even within a feeding session.

Lastly, infant formulas may have additives such as sugar to enhance their palatability and consequent marketability. The net result of these differences between infant formulas and breast milk is that they may conspire to defeat an infant's weak natural satiety mechanisms. As a result, bottle-fed babies may be more likely to overeat. The possibility that this may have repercussions in adulthood will be discussed below.

A possible link between infant overfeeding and adult fatness was suggested by reports on the effects of overfeeding on the development of fat cells. According to these reports, our total number of fat cells is established early in life. This number was thought to be increased by overfeeding. In adulthood we are left with our legacy of fat cells acquired in infancy. We can make these fat cells grow larger or smaller in size, but we cannot change their numbers. If it is true that fat cells generate a drive to fill themselves, then a large number of fat cells would produce a permanent tendency toward fatness.

This theory postulated that there were two fundamentally different types of fatness, *hyperplastic* and *hypertrophic*. Hyperplastic fatness is characterized by large numbers of fat cells. Since you cannot do anything about numbers of fat cells, hyperplastic fatness is very resistant to treatment. On the other hand, hypertrophic fatness is characterized by enlarged size as opposed to numbers of fat cells. Because fat-cell size can change, hypertrophic fatness may be more responsive to treatment.

The theory is extremely provocative because it implies a distinct fatalism toward fatness, at least with respect to the hyperplastic variety. In this sense it agrees with a genetic determinism in suggesting that if you have this sort of fatness, there is probably little you can do about it. It should be added that at present this theory is by no means proved. However, even if it is ultimately proved to be wrong, it will have created a stimulating controversy. And controversy is what this field needs, for at the moment, the prevailing mood is one of stultification and complacency.

GENDER

Males and females differ in both the total amount and distribution of their body fat. The body weight of a healthy young female is about 30 percent fat. A comparable male is only about

20 percent fat. Further, females have more of their fat just beneath the skin. This is why women tend to be more curvaceous than men.

Not only do females start out with more fat than males, they are also much more likely to accumulate excess fat. Survey after survey has shown that females are by far the more fat-afflicted sex. This is true at almost any age, in almost any culture. By any measure of fatness or weight, women are almost twice as likely as men to be too fat or too heavy.

The fat-proneness of women is important for at least two reasons. First, women are under the more social pressure to be thin (and therefore fashionable), yet women are generally far less successful at achieving thinness. Consequently, the psychological disturbances produced by failed attempts at dieting are much greater for women. Fat is very definitely a feminist issue.

The second point of importance concerns fat as a health hazard. Women are about twice as likely as men to be overweight yet they live substantially longer! This is completely at odds with the widespread view that obesity is one of the greatest health hazards of our time.

AGE

In general, the older you get, the fatter you get. The general increase in body weight levels off at around fifty with men, although women continue to get fatter for longer. Interestingly, by almost any measure, fatness seems to have been on the increase for at least the past thirty years in both men and women. At the same time, food intake appears to have decreased, and life expectancy has definitely increased. These findings have important implications for the issue of fatness as a health hazard (see chapter 2).

Numerous other social factors also have striking effects on the likelihood of becoming fat. The first four factors listed (i.e., heredity, early experience, gender, and age) suggest that in many cases there may not be much you can do to avoid getting fat. But there are other, more social and/or environmental factors also.

NATIONALITY

The prevalence of fatness varies widely among different ethnic and national groups. For example, North Americans of African descent are far more likely to be fat than those of European or Asian descent. This difference is mainly due to the extremely high proportion of fat black women. The ethnic differences in fatness among men are negligible. Native North Americans, particularly the Pima Indians of Arizona, are extremely fat. It would be very easy to conclude that the Pimas were simply genetically fat. However, this conclusion would be misleading, since obesity in the Pimas appears to have appeared only in quite recent times.

For thousands of years the Pimas cultivated crops under difficult conditions. Depending on the vagaries of the local climate, the availability of food fluctuated widely. Feast and famine were a regular part of the Pima way of life. As a consequence, Pimas are genetically geared to be good at getting fat in lush times and at conserving fat in hard times. Famine is now a thing of the past for the Pimas, but its legacy of physiological adaptations remains. The Pimas are "wired up" to get fat and to stay that way. In recent times of plenty that is just what they have done.

A rapid increase in fatness following a sudden shift from subsistence-level nutrition to a continuous supply of food has been seen in groups all around the world. It is interesting to note that the critical nutritional change is invariably not just one of quantity. These fat-promoting changes in nutrition always involve the introduction of high-fat and high-sugar foods along with the widespread use of alcohol. This, of course, means that whatever health liability these groups may incur is not simply due to their getting fat. Getting fat is only one element in a drastically changed nutritional and general health picture. How you get fat and stay fat may well be as important as the fatness itself. This potentially important nutritional-health issue has received little attention because of the almost exclusive emphasis on fat itself.

Although the ability to get fat may no longer be adaptive, it is by no means certain that it is necessarily maladaptive. In other words, it may not be particularly good to be fat, but it may not be all that bad. Certainly, the Pimas, for example, now show very high rates of diabetes. However, as pointed out above, it is not at all certain to what extent this is caused by the fatness as such. Their high-fat, high-sugar diet may be an important factor as well. The general obsession with fatness as the root of all health evils has impeded investigation in this direction. It is interesting that the longest life expectancy in the Pimas is found in those who are, by any standards, very fat. The fattest Pimas tend to be the healthiest Pimas. If, over the next few thousand years, the Pimas gradually regain their former slenderness, one could reasonably argue that their present fatness was maladaptive.

An energetic thriftness that can promote fatness certainly occurs in all human groups. However, the magnitude of this thriftiness varies greatly. For example, the men in Lagos, Nigeria, are among the most slender in the world in spite of an abundant and constant food supply. In contrast, the women in Lagos are very fat. Obesity is about eight times more common in the women. The men in Lagos are descendants of thousands of years of hunters. It is tempting to speculate that any weight gain in hunters (who are almost always men) would be very maladaptive.

Excess weight slows a hunter down, and most hunting methods rely heavily on speed. This means that hunters will have been subject to strong natural selection favoring those who are energetically wasteful. Being energetically wasteful greatly reduces the likelihood of becoming fat. In contrast, for men who are farmers and for most women, being able to move swiftly is of little advantage. For women and farmers, energetic thriftiness and the fatness it leads to would be distinct advantages because their extra fat would increase their resistance to the ravages of famine and disease.

A relative inability to gain weight is not simply an African male characteristic. Among the Bantus of southern Africa, the men are about as fat as their European and North American counterparts. However, once again the general rule applies that women are far more likely to be fat than men, and therefore Bantu women are considerably more likely to be fat than European or North American women.

Overall, national and ethnic groups vary widely in their fatness. Within these groups women are far more likely to be fat. These differences appear to reflect physiological characteristics that have evolved to deal with an environment that has changed radically. Whether these now obsolete physiological responses are simply irrelevant or are frankly maladaptive will take generations to determine. Meanwhile, there is some reason to believe that the general increase in fatness does not constitute some new plague visited upon us as a penalty for affluence.

The twentieth century is not the only period of long-term abundance of food in history. The abundance we enjoy may now be more widespread and affect a greater proportion of the population, but it is not a totally new state of affairs. If fatness were really catastrophic, it is likely that we would have developed physiological responses to prevent it. And, if this were the case, in times of prolonged abundance, physiological thriftiness should rapidly shift to physiological wastefulness. The slow, but progressive increase in the weight of humans indicates, however, that no such shift toward energetic wastefulness has occurred. Indirectly, this also suggests that fatness may not be so dangerous after all.

URBANIZATION

Another rather puzzling finding is that fatness appears to be strongly associated with the national level of urbanization. Country people are consistently fatter than their urban cousins. In rural Czechoslovakia the incidence of severe obesity is about three times as great as in urban Prague. The slenderizing effects of urbanization have been reported in many countries. These findings raise serious difficulties for traditional theories of fatness. Take, for example, the notion that fatness is due to eating too much junk food.

If the junk-food hypothesis of fatness were correct, country people would be less likely to be fat. Country areas usually have fewer junk-food outlets and fast-food emporiums. At the same time, country areas often have more available fresh produce. Both of these considerations suggest that, if excessive intake of "bad" foods is the culprit in fatness, then city dwellers should be fatter, not thinner, than country people.

On the other hand, if fatness is primarily due to inactivity, once again country people should be less likely to be fat, because country life is less automated than city life. This would suggest that simplistic notions based on the worship of exercise as the god that purges us of fatness may be on shaky grounds.

SOCIAL CLASS

The catchall category of social class encompasses religion, education, and status, as well as some of the variables discussed above. This area is filled with intriguing scraps of information, but making sense of these data is difficult. For example, Jews tend to be fatter than Catholics, and Catholics tend to be fatter than Protestants. You could make a stab at explaining this by saying that Jews are racially fatter or that their fatness reflects nationality differences. This explanation avoids the problem and is not really an explanation at all. The critical issue is, how do some groups get fat while others remain slim? Are Jews (or fat people in general) genetically programmed to eat more or to exercise less? Or is it something else altogether? Until this question is answered, we really haven't come closer to understanding fatness.

The problem of accounting for widely differing degrees of fatness in various ethnic groups is difficult when you compare groups such as Jews and Catholics who may also be racially different. However, these differences approach outright weirdness when you compare ethnic groups that are very similar on racial/national grounds. For example, among Protestants in the United States, Baptists are fatter than Methodists, and almost everyone is fatter than Episcopalians. Why the factors that determine fatness should differ in apparently similar groups is extremely puzzling. Surely these differences are not simply due to differences in food intake and exercise.

It is possible that these examples do not reflect true religious differences. They may instead be due to differences in urbanization. For instance, Baptists are more likely to live in the country than are Episcopalians. If, as I suspect, Methodists are intermediate in their level of urbanization, then the religious differences are obviously apparent, but not the determining factor. The real difference in fatness is due to urbanization. This begs the crucial question as to how urbanization, or anything else for that matter, causes changes in body weight.

A titillating possibility that may help to explain some of these differences is stress. Most people agree that increasing urbanization is associated with increasing degrees of stress. Ultimately, fatness is the expression of an energy imbalance (see chapter 4). When energy intake exceeds expenditure, the difference is stored as fat. Stress alters energy balance in two ways to produce fatness. It must increase food intake or decrease energy expenditure.

It is important to note that some stress-related hormones act as antagonists for insulin, the hormone whose deficiency is involved in diabetes (see chapter 2). This insulin antagonism can also reduce appetite. Stress may keep weight down by acting on both energy intake and energy expenditure. But stress can also predispose someone to developing diabetes. Should we then cultivate stress to keep our weight down? When put in these terms it seems clear that few would voluntarily opt for stress as a weight-reduction therapy.

There are all sorts of other 'natural'' weight-reducing aids. Smoking, drug addiction, depression, cancer, and tuberculosis are only a few. I think stress could be added to the above list. Stress is probably as unhealthy and dangerous a ''cure'' for fatness as are the others, yet unwittingly many dieters have chosen just this route.

Intelligent, well-educated people are much less likely to be fat than are less-advantaged people. This rather straightforward finding conceals a great deal of underlying complexity. One might be tempted to say that bright, educated people clearly see the folly of fatness and the virtues of slenderness. Even given this dubious basic assumption, we are once again left with the fundamental question as to how the anointed few achieve their salvation. Do they eat less, exercise more, or is it something else entirely?

The well-educated are more likely to be affluent. As a result, they may have ready access to more rich (i.e., fattening) foods. It doesn't seem likely that affluent people eat less than their less-affluent counterparts, however they may eat better. That is, the poor must often rely on cheap, energy-dense foods that are very high in saturated fats and simple sugars. It is possible that this peculiar dietary structure (and not simple calories) produces a tendency toward fatness. This explanation is made more plausible by the fact that it only occurs in developed countries. In poorer countries the poor people do not have the opportunity to be fat and that in these countries the rich tend to be fatter than the poor.

Affluent, educated people are less likely to expend a lot of energy in earning a living. The physical demands of menial jobs usually allotted to the poor should give them a head start in the battle against the bulge, yet, we have already discovered this is not the case. Once again, food intake and voluntary energy expenditure do not account for fatness. The effects of intelligence on a person's weight may be simply due to the fact that intelligent people are exposed to more stress. High-powered jobs are also high-stress jobs. Stress-induced increases in energy expenditure may be the "secret" to the slenderness of the affluent.

There is yet another reason why the rich and successful are thinner. It is an unsavory but undeniable fact of life that in the weight-obsessed countries of the West, fat people are actively discriminated against. This discrimination appears to be levied most strongly against women, but men are affected as well. Fat people do not have the same opportunities as the thin. (This is reflected in the fact that the "class" differences in body weight are much more pronounced in women than in men.) They are frequently denied access to career and educational opportunities that would improve their social position. Thus, the slenderness of the affluent may be an expression of unnatural selection.

What emerges from the present discussion may perhaps comfort the afflicted and afflict the comforted. Slenderness is widely viewed as a virtue on which the affluent have a special lease. On the other hand, fatness is widely viewed as a vice to which the dull and poor are particularly prone. The present analysis raises the possibility that the slenderness of the affluent may be a symptom of the price of being a high-achiever. Endemic slenderness is not a virtue—far from it. Instead, it may be a symptom of one of the most widespread and virulent diseases of our times: stress.

The foregoing analysis, heretical though it seems, is supported by evolutionary considerations. Throughout history, widespread slenderness has typically been the product of the ravages of famine or disease. During the period of human evolution, famine and disease have been the two omnipresent and universal stressors. As a result, it is not unreasonable that famine, whether it is self-inflicted or otherwise, may still mobilize other, less fashionable stress responses. Any long-term stress is almost certainly a health hazard. For the first time in history, millions of humans are voluntarily subjecting themselves to starvation stress. The irony of this is that perhaps one of the most tangible forms of progress is our ability to avoid the stress of starvation.

How Do You Get Fat?

Obesity is portrayed very simply as a disease of gluttony and sloth. It is assumed to be the result of overindulgence in food and underindulgence in exercise. These two assumptions are really the heart of our intense aversion to fatness. We will show here, and in chapter 3, that these assumptions are false. We will also show this loathing to be the prejudice that it is. An equally radical result of this reevaluation is that if fatness is not really due to gluttony and sloth in the first place, then dieting and exercise are not likely to be very much use in losing weight.

GLUTTONY

Do fat people overeat? This sounds like an easy question to answer, but it is not. The reason is that to measure food intake accurately requires virtually a prison environment in which a liquid diet is metered out periodically. This sort of coercive procedure itself would produce peculiar food intake. Given the choice, humans usually select a highly varied diet, of which liquids are a minor part.

What about the long-revered practice of counting calories? We can get the energy (caloric) value of various foods from tables found in many popular magazines. It should be relatively simple to give people carefully weighed amounts of food and to later weigh the leftovers. Even assuming that our subjects didn't cheat (a very naive and optimistic assumption), this procedure is not very satisfactory. The problem is that calorie tables are, at best, only rough approximations of the energy value of foods.

The energy value of even a relatively simple food such as an apple will vary considerably depending on the type of apple, its size, and freshness. The energy value of more complex foods such as meats may vary even more, depending on their fat and protein content. Two apparently similar pieces of meat may differ in their energy value by 50 percent. The net result of all these sources of variability is that calorie tables have so much error built into them they are not much use except to increase the weight of popular magazines.

It is doubtful whether even the most diligent use of calorie tables would allow you to estimate your true energy intake to within 10 percent. Although that may sound adequate, an error in energy balance of even 10 percent over a year could result in a 20 percent increase in weight. Since the great majority of weight-concerned humans are interested in relatively small (10 to 20 percent) amounts of weight that have accumulated over many years, calorie charts are not likely to tell us much about where their weight came from. They are not likely to differentiate the energy intake of fat and thin people.

That fatness is due to overeating is almost universally assumed, yet there is little evidence to support this most influential assumption. An equally important corollary is that excess weight can be effectively eliminated by undereating. There is little evidence to support the nearly universal assumption that diets work. In fact, there is an abundance of data showing that most fatness is not due to overeating and that diets rarely work.

SLOTH

If you conclude that fat people do not overeat, then you probably assume that inactivity is the real culprit. If fat people do not have a pathology of eating, they must have a pathology of activity. Fat people are generally believed to be sloths as well as gluttons. Inactivity is seen as compounding the fat produced by overeating. This superficially reasonable statement is actually very difficult to test, and again, available data do not support the popular belief.

These misconceptions actually obscure two quite distinct issues regarding the relationship between activity and fatness. These issues can be posed as separate questions: first, do people become fat due to a lack of exercise? Second, is exercise a good way to lose weight?

Because of technical difficulties associated with measuring activity, these questions are not easily researched or answered. Nevertheless, some rather important and heretical facts emerge from examining the literature. First of all, activity is only a fairly minor element in our total energy expenditure. All of the voluntary moving we do each day likely accounts for less than 10 percent of our total daily energy expenditure. In terms of looking for a culprit in producing fatness, these figures suggest that activity should not be a very prime suspect. Certainly, if someone were absolutely inactive and if their energy intake did not change at all, this 10 percent positive energy balance could lead to gross obesity.

The extreme condition of absolute inactivity does not normally occur, so the question becomes can lesser degrees of activity account for some people being fat and others being thin? The answer is that it is not very likely that differences in voluntary activity could have much of an impact on the occurrence of fatness. Although it is not likely, it is still a possibility. Therefore, we must consider the data on activity differences between fat and thin people.

As with many of the problems relating to fatness, the most precise data come from experimental investigations of laboratory animals. Some show that enforced physical inactivity may increase body fat in rats. It is not clear whether this increase in weight is due to underexercise as such, or whether it may instead be due to an increase in food intake. This latter mechanism is quite possible, since there are data showing that certain types of stress may increase food intake in rats. For a very active animal such as the rat, enforced inactivity could well be stressful. Earlier it was suggested that stress might have slenderizing effects, whereas here we are suggesting the opposite. This discrepancy may reflect the difference between acute and chronic stress. It may also reflect the fact that different stressors have different effects.

A more persuasive association between fatness and inactivity comes from demonstrations that genetically fat rats are less active than their normal-weight littermates and that the activity differences may appear before there are any differences in weight. Further, forced activity may reduce the excessive weight gain characteristic of genetically fat rats. However persuasive these data may at first appear, it would be premature to use them to support a role for inactivity in the development of fatness in humans.

One reason why the rat activity data should be applied with

great caution to humans concerns the relative role activity plays in the overall energy economy of the two species (see chapters 4 and 6). Because rats have a very high ratio of surface area to body weight, they use a lot of their energy maintaining a constant body temperature. Having a lot of surface area and a low volume makes them good radiators. Consequently, physical activity accounts for only a very small proportion of a rat's total energy expenditure.

The small contribution that activity makes to the energy economy of the rat is indicated by the fact that a 6-mile walk would only add about 3 percent to a rat's daily energy expenditure. On the other hand, in an elephant the relations are nearly reversed, with thermoregulation being relatively energetically "cheap" (they are bad radiators) and physical activity being "expensive." A 6-mile walk would add over 20 percent to the energy expenditure of an elephant.

These figures mean that even if a rat took a daily 6-mile constitutional, it would have only a small effect on its overall energy balance. In contrast, the same stroll would have a large effect on the energy economy of an elephant. Whenever activity is implicated as a major factor in regulating the weight of rats, one can safely bet that the effect is not due to activity as such but to some other factor in the energy-balance equation. The data, then, do not suggest that inactivity as such is a major factor in the development of fatness in rats. On the more positive side, you can safely bet that a slothful elephant is a fat elephant.

Energetically speaking, humans fall between rats and elephants. We are only moderately good radiators of heat, consequently physical activity is a moderately important element in our overall energy economy. For example, a 6-mile walk would likely increase our total energy expenditure by about 10 percent. As mentioned above, a 10 percent reduction in energy expenditure could lead to fatness if all other things were equal. The problem is that all other things are almost never equal. A reduction in activity is likely to lead to a reduction in food intake. Similarly, increases in activity often produce compensatory increases in food intake. There are other, still more complex changes in the overall energy economy that can further obscure the relation between activity and fatness (see chapter 6).

All of this is still largely theoretical. It does not directly address the original question of whether fat people are less active. Even that question is not directly what we are interested in, which is whether inactivity leads to fatness. Fat people may just be inactive because they are fat. Particularly in very fat people, even rather simple movements can be quite difficult. This is a major disadvantage of being really fat. This fundamental question whether inactivity is a cause of fatness or a result of it seems to go largely ignored.

There are virtually no good data that show fat people are less active than their lean counterparts. For every study that has claimed to show a positive relation between inactivity and fatness, there are at least two that show no such relation. Further, even the best of the positive data are not very compelling.

One of the most widely cited studies purporting to show that fatness has its roots in sloth used cinematography to investigate activity in adolescent girls. Any scholarly work on exercise and body weight is certain to cite this landmark study in which two groups of fat and thin girls were filmed playing sports during their stay at a summer camp. This technique presents a combination of relatively high-tech data acquisition and low-tech data analysis. It seems to have captured the imagination of most of the liniment fraternity. The results showed that fat, adolescent girls were less active during sports than their thin counterparts. The fact that this finding is essentially meaningless has gone unnoticed.

There are several reasons why these data are meaningless. One is that the fat and thin girls were at different camps. In other words, differences in the activity could be linked more to the camps than the issue of fatness/thinness. The relative lethargy of the fat girls could well reflect the coercive nature of the exercise used in their camp. Or, since the purpose of the camp was to get the girls to lose weight, the apparent lethargy of the fat girls could reflect the debiliating effects of the strict dieting that was inflicted upon them. Another possibility is that the fat girls could well have been sent to the camp by their parents because they were particularly inactive in the first place. There are still other reasons why these data are likely meaningless, but the above should be quite enough.

CHAPTER 2

FEAR OF FAT

The widespread misinformation given about the relation of fatness to health is a reflection of what a shoddy state the fat business is in. Health authorities elbow each other off stage in their zeal to warn the public of the dangers of fat. Hardly a weekend newspaper goes by without the usual pious warnings of the doom visited upon those who refuse to purge themselves of the sin of fatness. Fat has become a matter of sin and retribution. The moral overtones of the fear of fat are inescapable. Thin people see themselves as morally superior because they are not only beautiful but healthy as well. Conversely, they look upon the willful ugliness and unhealthiness of fat people as a sign of their moral inferiority. The aesthetic inferiority of fatness is arbitrary. The unhealthfulness of fatness has been badly overstated. Fat is not a moral issue.

FUELING OUR PHOBIAS

At one time or another fat people have been said to be the special prey of practically every known disease and to live brief and blighted existences. Incorrect views as to the dangers of fatness continue to dominate both professional and public attitudes in spite of their lack of validity. The prevalent fear and loathing of fatness is unjustified and also dangerous.

The inadequacy of the portrayal of fatness as a toxic condition begins with the nature of the data used to support this view. Much of the best-publicized evidence for the idea that fatness is a health hazard comes from actuarial data provided by American life insurance companies. These data, which will be discussed in some detail below, have been badly misinterpreted. They do not support the blanket condemnation that comes from the antifat activists. Since the fatophobes have had the ear of the public for some time, the public has come to believe their gospel. It is now widely accepted as self-evident that fatness is a disease that endangers us all. The public has, as yet, had little exposure to the heresy you are now reading. Fatness is rarely a disease, and it is very often not at all dangerous.

The antifat lobby has paid little attention to the validity of the evidence they use to support their cause. Most of this evidence is so indirect and equivocal that it renders their conclusions unwarranted. The condemnation of fat as a major health menace is based upon a misinterpretation of the available data. At the same time, it requires ignoring the considerable body of evidence that points to quite different, even opposite conclusions. This conspicuous lack of enlightenment is particularly dangerous because much of it comes from august sources. Almost everyone believes that fat is one of the greatest health hazards of our time, which leads in turn to an irrational fear of it. Where there is fear, loathing is not far behind. Fear and loathing of fat have become an integral part of most of our lives. This destructive attitude is buttressed by both medical and folk wisdom. This widespread support does not justify these views. It does, however, make them dangerous.

The misrepresentation of the relation of fatness to health is not just idle quackery. It has harmful effects on both fat and thin people and it undermines the credibility of the medical profession. Physicians have been fighting a battle against all sorts of "alternative" medicines on the often-defensible grounds that they are ultimately unhealthy. The danger in alternative medicine lies not simply in the fact that it doesn't work. Using nonmedical medicine often prevents people from obtaining conventional medical help that could really work. Further, quack therapies often minimize or even prevent an unbiased evaluation of their effectiveness. An objective assessment of the effectiveness of any treatment is essential to separating the wheat from the chaff. Alternative medicines are often pure and simple obscurantism. In the long run nobody profits from obscurantism. This is why the subject of fatness is buried in chaff.

With respect to fatness, much of the medical profession is engaged in the implicit or explicit support of the same sort of snake medicine that it vigorously opposes in other arenas. It is an encouraging sign that there is an increasing number of physicians who no longer subscribe to the antiquated views of fat that still prevail in the marketplace. A more realistic and optimistic view of the role of fat in health is gradually emerging. However, these revisionist attitudes are being fought tooth and nail. Some opponents of these views are well intentioned, but misinformed. Others are interested in preserving the status quo for purely commercial reasons. Fat is big business.

The issue of body weight is one of the rare fields where mainstream medicine and various "antimedicines" often become indistinguishable. In this case, antimedicine does not care about data, and much of mainstream medicine continues to settle for second-rate and seriously misinterpreted data. This strange alliance is partially due to the fact that neither mainstream nor alternative medicine offers any real cure to combat fatness. However, the nonprescription antidotes foisted upon a gullible and frightened public have all sorts of ugly repercussions. Like other misguided treatments, they are not only ineffective, they are ultimately harmful. Alternative medicine may be just the thing for alternative health problems, but it is of no use to those who are afflicted with conventional health problems. As yet, I have not heard of an alternative health problem.

The negative effects of this obsession are painfully apparent. Eating disorders, particularly in women, have reached epidemic proportions (see chapter 8). Eating disorders are just one aspect of the ill health that results from a continual and futile battle against one's own body. Misunderstandings about what can and should be done about fat are a source of great unhappiness to millions.

Those who try to lose weight and fail are held to be weak and immoral by the community at large. Even worse, they frequently develop a contempt for themselves. The self-hatred so common among failed dieters is a reflection of irrational public attitudes toward fatness. The category of failed dieters includes at least 95 percent of those who have ever attempted to lose weight. Fat people soon learn that there is little they can do about their weight. Since they are repeatedly told that their fat is the source of all their woes, many come to believe that they are powerless. The feeling of loss of control over one's own fate is one of the most psychologically destructive afflictions known. It is a central element in psychiatric disorders such as depression and anxiety, as well as being a contributory factor in countless other physical and psychological problems. This assault is as needless as it is harmful.

Mortality and Body Weight

The core of the health argument is that fat people are more prone to all sorts of diseases. The bottom line of the argument is that fat people are said to die young. While there is some truth in this statement, the picture is not nearly as dismal as we are usually told as we will see below. However, even if the statement were absolutely and unequivocally true, the corrective action suggested is something else entirely. For this fact to be used legitimately in the advocacy of weight loss, it must be shown that it is the fatness that causes the early death. It would be absurd to deny that some fat people have a marked health liability. However, it is often questionable whether this liability is due to being fat as such. The relatively poor health status of fat people reflects the action of a number of risk factors of which fat is only one. Excessive emphasis on fat as the root of ill health is dangerous since fat is often the most intractable of a constellation of risk factors.

When people find that they can do little about their fat, they frequently abandon all hope of being able to maintain their own health. The pressures to lose weight are enormous. They are buttressed by misleading information on the role of fat in health and by an extraordinary set of aesthetic prejudices. Since the physician's "medicine" to bring about weight loss is almost certainly ineffective, it is not surprising that many patients simply lose faith in their physician and in medicine as a whole. This sort of nihilism is extremely unhealthy.

The erroneous views are mainly based on life insurance data. The Build and Blood Pressure Study pooled data from over 4 million life insurance policies issued in the United States between 1935 and 1954. The data consisted of age, height, weight, and blood pressure. The mortality rates in the various groups suggested that the lighter you are, the better. This interpretation was naive even by the standards of the 1950s. There are a number of reasons why the bleak picture they painted was not valid then, and is even less valid now.

The analysis and interpretation of medical data have come a long way since the 1950s. It is most unfortunate that these improvements have not been reflected in current views about the role of fatness in health. Although a reasonable interpretation of these data is available, it does not appear to have reached the ears of the general public. Even many health professionals appear to be unaware that it is no longer the 1950s. The continuing misinformation is doing all of us harm.

One problem with life insurance data is that they are based on a highly selected group of people. The more this group differs from the general population, the less applicable the conclusions are to anyone else. The vast majority of life insurance policies on which the Build and Blood Pressure Study based its conclusions were issued to a group that is not at all representative of the general public. The insurance policies were held by upper-middle-class Anglo-Saxon males who lived in cities in the northeastern United States. Moreover, the insured men were substantially lighter than the rest of the population in the first place. These men were not at all representative of even white, male urban Americans, let alone the rest of the world. We will see below that the conclusions were not even valid for the target group.

To use data from such a nonrepresentative group to estimate the effect of fatness on the health of people in general is utter foolishness. Yet this is just what is being done. The life insurance data are presented as showing essentially universal relationships between fatness and health. It is becoming increasingly apparent that data from highly selected groups do not allow such broad generalizations.

Even to use the life insurance data to infer the role of fatness in the health of other Americans in the northeastern United States is probably not justified. In fact, because relatively few people owned life insurance policies thirty years ago, this group may not even be representative of upper-middle-class, white male urban underweight northeastern Americans. People who held life insurance even thirty years ago were a very select group. This is probably not as true of life insurance policy holders now, but it certainly was then.

Just how different insured people may be from the rest of the population is shown by an analysis of deaths in women in the middle and late nineteenth century. Women who were insured died younger! On the basis of this information one could conclude that life insurance is a health hazard or that the insured women were not representative of women in general. It is likely that the latter is true. One way the insured women differed was that more of them were married. Is marriage a health hazard for women? A more likely explanation is that mortality during childbirth was much higher in the nineteenth century, and most children were born to married women. Similarly, the husbands of these women were astute observers of the chances of their spouses living long lives. The point is that a superficial analysis yields conclusions that have superficial validity at most. Popular interpretations of the role of fatness in health tend to be both superficial and misleading.

The central confusion lies in the difficulty of isolating the negative effects of fatness *per se* from all the other differences between fat and nonfat people. Since groups of fat people often have a greater health liability than comparable groups of nonfat people, it is important to determine whether fatness actually causes the liability. Fatness could merely be a symptom of another process that causes the ill health instead of being the cause of ill health itself. If, as would seem likely, fat itself often does not cause ill health and premature death, a lot of people have been barking up the wrong tree. Further, if fat is not the real culprit, losing weight might not be expected to have any dramatic health benefits.

To express this another way, it would not be surprising if people who wore multiple earrings had a shorter life expectancy than those who wore no earrings. This positive relation between earring wearing and early death would likely be due to the fact that multiple-earring wearers typically have a more than usually dangerous life-style. Would it be correct to say that earrings are a health hazard? If a public education program entirely eradicated earring wearing, would anyone be any healthier?

There is good reason to believe that the relation between fatness and health is not all that different from earring wearing and health.

Fatness is a common complication of both diabetes and high blood pressure. That is, these disorders may actually cause fatness as opposed to being the result of it. The situation is somewhat similar in the case of hyperlipidemia. The latter condition is most commonly seen as elevated cholesterol levels. There is little dispute that these diseases are potential killers. For this reason alone, fat people would be expected to have a higher-than-normal mortality rate. In these cases, however, the real culprit is the diabetes, hypertension, and hyperlipidemia. It is clear that weight loss often reduces the symptoms of all these disorders, but it is by no means clear that weight gain causes any of them. At most, the current evidence suggests that weight gain may precipitate diabetes and hypertension, though there appears to be little evidence that weight gain as such precipitates hyperlipidemia. The problem is that weight gain is often associated with high fat intake, which can precipitate and exacerbate hyperlipidemia. If you have warning signs or a family history of these conditions, weight gain is to be avoided. However, this commonsense advice tends to overlook the fact that it is often exceedingly difficult for these very people to maintain a "safe" body weight.

From the inarguable base of the salutary effects of weight loss in diabetics, hypertensives, and hyperlipidemics, it is commonly argued that weight loss will also benefit all fat people. There are those who have taken this error still further and maintain that even nonfat people should lose weight. This is an unhealthy distortion of a simple truth. There is no good evidence that weight loss is at all beneficial for the vast majority of overweight people without these diseases. There is even less evidence that slimming would improve the health of those who are not fat.

The indiscriminate advocacy of weight loss is often said to be supported by another piece of the life insurance data. An analysis of data from the 1940s uncovered a group who lost weight during the period between the issuing of successive policies. This group had a longer life expectancy than a group who had not lost weight during the same period. This is the only piece of evidence even suggesting that weight loss increases life expectancy in the general population. As we will show below, this interpretation is not justified.

Quite apart from the fact that life insurance data say relatively little about the general population, there are other errors in this analysis. For example, if weight losers were prompted to lose weight by virtue of their having diabetes, hypertension, and/or hyperlipidemia, then, of course, their life expectancy would be improved. A large group is certain to contain a substantial number of people with these disorders. Certainly, weight loss is good medicine for selected groups in the population. However, this says nothing about any potential benefits for nondiseased fat people or nonfat people. For diabetics, hypertensives, and hyperlipidemics, weight loss is a highly desirable goal. These people should be encouraged to attempt to lose weight. However, it is quite wrong to suggest on the basis of such findings that weight loss is good medicine for most, or even many people.

Another important deficiency of these data can be seen when comparing the two groups on points other than weight loss. If these people were concerned enough about their health to lose weight, they probably changed their life-styles in other important respects as well. Health-conscious people rarely smoke and usually drink in moderation. Further, they usually exercise regularly and eat a healthy diet. Lastly, they usually have regular medical examinations. These examinations would certainly lead to the diagnosis of any danger signs at a stage when they could more easily be dealt with. It would be very surprising if such sweeping improvements in life-style did not lead to some overall increase in life expectancy. To the essential question of whether the increased longevity is due to the weight loss, the answer is no. These data do not implicate weight loss as the cause of increased longevity.

There is another possibility that could account for the improved life expectancy of the group who lost weight: This group may not have been comparable with the others in the first place. We will see in chapters 5 through 7 that an exceedingly small proportion of the population can permanently lose weight. Successful weight losers are very exceptional. They could well be so different from the general population that their life expectancy would be longer irrespective of their weight loss. This is not mere sophistry. People who are successful at weight loss are even less representative of the population as a whole than are insurance policy holders. The fact that the people in question were both weight losers and policy holders makes them very unusual indeed.

There is no evidence suggesting that weight loss will improve the health of people in general. More damning yet, there is quite a lot of evidence suggesting that, excepting extreme emaciation or obesity, body weight *by itself* has relatively little impact on health or life expectancy. The vast majority of data showing the inferior health status of fat people ignore the obvious fact that fat people are different from nonfat people in many other ways besides their fatness. These other differences invariably turn out to be more important as health liabilities than the fat itself. In other words, a great many people who are worried about their fat as a health hazard are unnecessarily concerned. This needless concern is stressful. Stress is a health hazard. What are we doing to each other?

It would be a gross and dangerous misinterpretation of this book if genuinely endangered fat people used it as an excuse for avoiding what could be good medicine for them. Diabetics, hypertensives, and hyperlipidemics can improve their health by losing weight. This point should not be lost in these arguments. The practicality of this suggestion is an entirely different issue from its desirability. Weight loss is undoubtedly desirable for some people, but it is an attainable goal for very few. The fact that weight loss is so difficult to achieve does not mean that, for those who really need it, it should not be attempted. The problem is that the attitudes about fat are so obsessional that other forms of probably more effective and practical treatments are often lost in the shuffle. Further, apart from causing ill health, irrational attitudes about what we should and can do with our bodies are impoverishing the lives of millions.

The best way to determine the effects of body weight on longevity is to examine the entire population and not just an unrepresentative group such as those who take out life insurance. Since this leviathan undertaking is unlikely to be done, we must settle for approximations of the ideal study. These compromise studies must investigate groups that are reasonably representative of the whole population. Fortunately, there are a few studies like this, the results of which lead to very different conclusions from those in general circulation.

The most famous of these studies is the Framingham Study. This classic study enlisted about half the people between thirty and sixty years of age in Framingham, Massachusetts. Although this sample of about five thousand people was smaller than the insurance company sample, it was much more representative of the American population. The Framingham group received regular medical examinations, and the causes of the deaths in these people were carefully recorded over a number of years. The highest mortality rate was found in the thinnest men! A prominent socialite once said, "It's impossible to be too rich or too thin." She was, at best, half right.

Extreme thinness is associated with ill health. Extremes of nearly every physiological condition are markers of ill health. People who are physiologically exceptional in one respect will probably be exceptional in other respects as well. To isolate one characteristic and say that it is the only cause of ill health is unjustified. There could be some justification for such a leap beyond the available data if there were sound theoretical reasons why such a finding might occur. There are some reasons why fatness might be harmful to health, but they are not very compelling. More important, the data do not paint the frightening picture of the consequences of fatness that we are told about.

The indictment of thinness provided by the Framingham Study is virtually the opposite of what the life insurance companies repeatedly claim are immutable and universal truths. It is more than a little curious that crusaders against fatness tend to overlook this aspect of the study. Why are there not people beating the bushes crying, "Woe to the thin, the end is near"? Thin people are never accused of lacking willpower or self-control. Junk-food emporiums could advertise themselves as the true health food centers. Of course this is silly, but it is no more silly than the pious twaddle that is regularly inflicted on fat people.

The essential picture to emerge from the Framingham Study is that being either very thin or very fat is associated with a reduced life expectancy. This does not come as a great surprise, since it is basically common sense. Yet, common sense has been all too rare in this area. However, the real punch line of the Framingham Study is that, apart from the two extremes, body weight has very little effect on mortality! This finally suggests a useful definition of *ideal weight*. An ideal weight is one that is more than sepulchral thinness and less than gross obesity. This definition has at least as much validity as any of the others. It further means that most of the population is already at an ideal weight.

Fat and Your Heart

The main thrust of the argument that asserts fatness increases mortality is that fatness is bad for your heart. The fear of heart disease has millions counting calories and pounding the pavement. "Eat properly, exercise regularly, and lose weight" is the litany describing the path to a healthy heart. The first two of these prescriptions are sound advice. Unfortunately, the third verse of the litany probably undoes much of the benefit that could be produced by the others. The reason is simple. It is relatively easy for most people to eat properly and to exercise, and such practices can be of some benefit to almost everyone. The situation with weight is very different. First, it is nearly impossible for most people to lose weight (see chapters 5 through 7). In addition, weight loss would likely benefit relatively few people. Equally important is the fact that a great many people who fail at weight loss throw in the towel and abandon other, easily attainable health objectives. This is not a trivial problem, since at least 95 percent of dieters fail miserably. An excessive emphasis on the importance of weight to cardiovascular health is an unhealthy practice.

There are three main reasons why fat is believed to endanger the heart. The most common one is that any excess weight overworks the heart. The next reason is that fatness produces problems with blood lipids, such as cholesterol. The damage to the blood vessels produced by high cholesterol is thought to lead to other, more direct forms of heart disease. Lastly, many believe that the effects of fatness on the heart are secondary to the high blood pressure caused or exacerbated by fatness. We will consider the three arguments individually below. It turns out that each of them is seriously flawed. The errors in these arguments are not simply minor academic nit-picking. They are sufficiently great to say that the impact of fatness on cardiovascular health has been greatly exaggerated. Again, this is not to say that fatness is good for the heart or that some fat people should not lose weight. It does, however, mean that a great many people are needlessly worried about what their body weight is doing to their heart.

It is a common notion that fatness strains the heart and that this overwork leads to its premature demise. Being fat is depicted as the physiological equivalent of overloading one's car. This logic may be valid for cars, but it is not generally valid for people. It may well apply to those rare unfortunates who are massively obese, but to infer any effects from these rare pathologies to fat people in general is not justified. Exercise is a form of straining the cardiovascular system, yet most believe that exercise is good for the heart.

The notion that fat creates problems with blood lipids such as cholesterol is a much more plausible notion. Here the real culprit may well be the intake of saturated fats and not fatness per se. There are well-described means by which elevated cholesterol levels can cause damage to blood vessels, which in turn can cause all sorts of dangerous changes. For example, cholesterol is involved in the formation of atherosclerotic plaque, which narrows blood vessels. This narrowing increases the resistance to blood flow and elevates blood pressure. High blood pressure can itself cause damage to the walls of the blood vessels. This damage can serve as a focus for atheroslcerosis (see below). To appreciate this fully requires a brief discussion of the relation of cholesterol to other blood lipids.

Lipids such as cholesterol are not soluble in water. Their insolubility means that they have to be transported in the blood by special carrier molecules called lipoproteins. There are two fundamentally different types of lipoprotein. *Low-density lipoprotein (LDL)* transports cholesterol and triglycerides (see "Fat Is Your Friend," in chapter 1) to various target sites in the body. At these sites, the lipids are normally used immediately or stored for later use. *High-density lipoprotein (HDL)* may be thought of as a lipid scavenger. HDLs pick up lipids in the blood and carry them to the liver. The liver breaks down the lipids, and they are ultimately excreted.

There are at least a couple of ways that lipids can cause vascular problems. First, with extremely high levels of dietary intake of fats, lipids begin to accumulate in the arteries. The accumulation occurs because the HDLs can no longer handle the cleaning-up chores. The resultant arterial accumulation of lipids is known as *atherosclerosis*. It is interesting that cholesterol in the blood may only be minimally affected by dietary intake of cholesterol. This is because the liver's production of cholesterol adjusts itself to maintain a relatively constant level of blood cholesterol. High cholesterol levels are likely to be secondary with impaired handling of lipids. This can be brought about by high intake of saturated fats, but dietary intake of cholesterol itself may be fairly unimportant.

The second cause of atherosclerosis is both more common and more insidious. From time to time, arteries may suffer minor structural damage. Normally, this damage heals quite quickly. However, in some cases, the damage may act as a focal point for the accumulation of lipids. The reasons for this tendency are still disputed, but the existence of the effect is well established. Moreover, it is not at all certain why some people are very prone to atherosclerosis, whereas others are practically immune to it. Sometimes atherosclerosis is not even a result of arterial damage. Simple blood turbulence may be enough to create an atherosclerotic focus.

Irrespective of how it starts, once there is an initial accumulation of lipids, the process is likely to become a vicious circle. Atherosclerosis is particularly dangerous since it is often not detected until it is well advanced. One important sign of impending atherosclerosis is high levels of blood cholesterol. Cholesterol tests have become a routine part of medical examinations because they are a marker of impaired handling of lipids. Anything that has an unfavorable effect on blood lipids is a health hazard. It is widely assumed that fatness has such an unfavorable effect. Thus the argument implicating fatness in cardiovascular health seems plausible. Of course, plausibility does not make it correct. In the final analysis what really matters is the data. We will consider the data for this hypothesis below, after discussing the logic of the association between fatness and high blood pressure.

Although fatness is often associated with high blood pressure, there is no very plausible mechanism to account for such an association. It is obvious how hypertension can cause vascular problems, but it is not obvious how fatness can cause hypertension. The correlations between fatness and high blood pressure are fairly strong, but apart from that the picture is very unclear. This should not be so surprising, since the causes of high blood pressure are far from being agreed upon either in fat or in thin people. Fortunately, this has not prevented the development of several effective forms of treatment for high blood pressure. One of these treatments is weight loss.

The association between fatness and high blood pressure is fairly compelling. High blood pressure is prevalent in developed, fat societies and it is very rare in undeveloped, thin ones. Also, rapid weight gain in young adults is a strong danger sign for the development of high blood pressure. There are, however, several lines of evidence suggesting that fatness may not necessarily cause high blood pressure. Perhaps the most obvious is that there are many fat people who have perfectly normal blood pressure. In addition, although weight loss often reduces blood pressure, it is not an invariable effect.

The lack of a causal relation between fatness and high blood pressure is further indicated by findings that people with high blood pressure are more prone to weight gain than those who do not have high blood pressure. In this light, high blood pressure and fatness would be seen as symptoms of a separate factor. It is important to note that successful therapy does not require a precise knowledge of causal relations. The effectiveness of any treatment is the important thing. Given an effective treatment, it is then up to the laboratory scientists to find out why the treatment works. For this reason alone, weight loss could be seen as desirable for anyone with high blood pressure.

The above arguments are essentially theoretical. The lack of a plausible mechanism for translating fatness into heart disease is academic if fatness can be shown to be bad for the heart. Whether or not fat is bad for the heart can be answered in several ways. The most common approach to this problem is to examine epidemiological studies such as the Framingham Study. There are other more direct ways as well. We will see below that the evidence used by the antifat lobby does not support their conclusions. Fat is nothing like the cardiovascular health hazard that most people believe it to be. Nor is fat totally innocuous with respect to cardiovascular health.

There are major deficiencies in the arguments on which the condemnation of fat is based. The deficiencies of these old arguments are not secret nor are they trivial. They have been outlined in detail in numerous respectable publications. Unfortunately, many antifat crusaders have made up their minds and use only data that support their conclusions. They ignore the mass of data that does not support or frankly refutes their conclusions. This is not good science or medicine. It is dangerous quackery. This gerrymandering of the truth has helped to make weight loss one of the most active hunting grounds for charlatans. Distorted views as to what fat means and what one should do about it form the basis of this charlatanism.

The Framingham Study remains useful because it is typical of what is good and bad about others of its type. Superficially, the Framingham data suggest that fatness is bad for the heart. This is almost the only aspect of the Framingham Study that the antifat lobby likes to talk about. However, even at a superficial level, there are numerous flies in the ointment, suggesting that all is not well with the conventional interpretation. When the data are examined more critically, the conventional interpretation becomes quite untenable.

One important aspect of the data that the antifat lobby usually ignores is the fact that the increased risk from being fat *decreases* with age. This is the opposite of what should happen if fatness were a degenerative disease. There is also a circulatory problem of the lower limbs, called intermittent claudication, which is *less* likely to occur in fat people. Fatness appears to be a protection against this form of vascular disease. This is interesting since the conventional wisdom is that fat people should be more prone to circulatory problems (see below). Other data also show that fat people are less likely to suffer from tuberculosis and suicide. Should we then conclude that slenderness cause intermittent claudication, tuberculosis, and suicide? Of course not; and complementary condemnation of fatness may be similarly unjustified.

A closer analysis of the Framingham Study leads to very different conclusions from those that appear in the popular press. In order to make sense of these data, one must take into account a variety of important differences between fat and lean people other than their weight. The Framingham Study included measures of a number of risk factors, such as smoking, blood pressure, and serum cholesterol. These variables make it possible to conduct a multivariate analysis. A multivariate analysis allows the specification of the independent effects of each of the variables. Typical analyses simply lump all the variables together. To attribute any complex effect to any one variable is quite incorrect unless the statement is based on a multivariate analysis. Unfortunately, this sort of fundamental procedural error remains commonplace in both the popular and scientific literature about fat.

Since smoking, blood pressure, and serum cholesterol all have their own effects on heart disease, it is important to distinguish their effects from those of fatness by itself. The multivariate analysis of the Framingham Study indicates that body weight *by itself* has no effect on cardiovascular disease, no effect on brain infarction, a slight positive effect on congestive heart failure in women only, and a slight positive effect on coronary heart disease. These effects are statistically significant, but they are quite small. This distinction between statistical significance and medical significance will be further considered below. Even if accepted uncritically, the Framingham Study is far from being the blanket condemnation of fatness that many claim it to be.

It has been said that the importance of the multivariate analysis is largely academic, since fatness does not act as an independent variable. For example, weight loss often produces a drop in blood pressure and lipids as well. This suggests that weight loss may influence other variables in such a way as to improve cardiovascular health. In this case, the precise causality does not really matter. This alone means that weight loss is good medicine for those with high blood pressure. This important fact should not be obscured. However, the strength of the advocacy of weight loss must be tempered by its practicality. We will see in chapter 5 that weight loss is achieved by only a tiny percentage of those who attempt it. Telling many people to lose weight to control their blood pressure may be like telling schizophrenics to "pull themselves together." It may well be desirable, but if it is not possible, it is not very useful advice.

Critics of the multivariate interpretation of the Framingham Study have said that it may not have painted a sufficiently bleak picture of the role of fatness in cardiovascular health because it did not follow the subjects long enough. If fatness is a malignant disorder, its effects might only become obvious over a longer period of time. At any rate, it would be useful to have follow-up data on the Framingham subjects. There are now such data. These data are widely interpreted as finally providing the missing link (that is, conclusive data) that the health community has been looking for.

There must have been a general sigh of relief among the antifat crusaders when they read the follow-up of the Framingham data. There in bold print was the verdict: "Obesity is an Independent Risk Factor for Cardiovascular Disease." This long-awaited proof is supported by highly significant statistics. Without disputing the banner statement, its import for the overall view of the role of fatness in cardiovascular health is surprisingly small. To understand why statistically significant results may have little medical significance requires some explanation.

The long awaited verdict was that "Obesity is an Independent Risk Factor for Cardiovascular Disease," but the latest interpretation of the Framingham data confuses statistical significance and medical-scientific significance. These are entirely separate issues. Statistical regression coefficients provide two pieces of information about relations among events. The statistical significance of a regression coefficient tells us whether the relationship observed would be likely to happen by chance. A chance happening is of little importance. The major relationships reported in the above study were clearly not simply chance occurrences. For example, after the twenty-six-year follow-up, the regression coefficient between weight and coronary heart disease was significant beyond the $p<0.001$ level. This means that chance factors would be expected to produce such a relationship in less than one out of a thousand cases.

The high statistical significance of the coefficient was interpreted as indicating that the relationship is both powerful and important. However, several considerations suggest that this relationship is not at all powerful or important. The value of the coefficient on which their momentous conclusion was based is a tiny 0.012. The only reason a figure this small even approaches statistical significance is because of the large number of observations involved. This sort of statistical significance is largely an artifact of having so many observations. Elementary statistical textbooks caution against this sort of artifact. However, the dubious nature of the statistical significance of these coefficients is not their most serious deficiency.

The most important characteristic of regression coefficients is what they tell us about the strength or predictive power of relationships. For example, it is possible for two variables to be correlated in a highly significant manner but if the correlation is small, the importance of the relationship would be minimal. The predictive power of regression coefficients is determined by converting them into a figure that expresses the amount of the variability in the relationship they explain. This is done by squaring the coefficient. For example, a coefficient of 0.900 would account for 81 percent of the variability, and 0.500 would account for 25 percent of the variability. As the coefficients get smaller, their predictive value diminishes very rapidly. A coefficient of 0.100 only accounts for 1 percent of the variability.

In the Framingham data, the highest regression coefficient between weight and coronary heart disease was 0.012. Squaring 0.012 indicates that this correlation accounts for about 0.01 percent of the observed variability! One one-hundredth of 1 percent is such a minuscule proportion of the variability as to be functionally medically insignificant. The coefficient is statistically significant, but it is practically devoid of any predictive power. This is not what we are told. These data may show that increased body weight is an independent cardiovascular risk factor, but it is definitely a minor one. It is not the sort of risk that should engender this state of near panic.

There are even more direct data suggesting that the case for the dangers of fatness to cardiovascular health has been overstated. To make this point more accessible, I will only discuss coronary artery disease. It is the most prevalent form of heart disease and has been strongly associated with atherosclerosis. The question is whether fatness causes either coronary heart disease or atherosclerosis.

For example, Metropolitan Life Insurance data suggest that the death rate from cardiovascular disease in fat men was 150 percent that of men who were not fat. In airline pilots, fatness was found to be a good predictor of sudden death and myocardial infarction. More recently, the American Cancer Society found a strong association between weight and subsequent cardiovascular death. These data are the very foundations of the fear of fat. Multicolor graphs depicting these gruesome results adorn countless brochures issued by public health authorities and weight-loss businesses. The people who distribute this information do not mention that these frightening statistics are not representative of a much larger body of information that points to different, even opposite conclusions.

In the classic Seven Countries Study, fat men were *less* likely to die from cardiovascular disease. The same finding has also been reported in men from southern Europe. In Finland, where cardiovascular disease is extremely prevalent, the men in the top 10 percent of the weight distribution were shown to have the lowest incidence of cardiovascular disease. Further, even in the United States, it is well known that mortality from cardiovascular disease has been decreasing steadily, whereas fatness has been increasing. Another study compared 866 American soldiers who died of coronary causes with a similar group who died of various accidental causes. The two groups showed no differences in fatness either at the time of admission to the army or at the time of death. All of these findings are the opposite of the conventional view that fat is little less than a bullet to the heart. It would not be honest to report the latter studies as portraying typical or universal relationships because there are other studies that suggest still different associations. However, it is not honest to report the few positive studies as portraying immutable and important relationships. Unfortunately, this lack of fundamental honesty in reporting data is all too common. Ignorance is no longer an adequate excuse.

Part of the reason for the differences in the relations described in the above studies is that they are drawn from very different groups. This suggests that the danger of fatness for the heart is modified by numerous social and racial factors. Even in very homogeneous groups, the relation between fatness and cardiovascular health is not what the health-through-thinness zealots tell us it is. One study of over twelve thousand white, middle-aged American men showed that fatness was only a cardiovascular risk in those who were at least 30 percent overweight. However, even among the six subgroups that made up this study, there were major differences. Several groups showed the effect and several others did not. Clearly, cardiovascular health is determined by a great many factors. Body weight is one of them, but it is probably not a major one. Weight has received more attention than it is due simply because it is deceivingly easy to point at and measure. Many of the other variables are not obvious and are much more difficult to measure.

The most direct way of investigating the effects of fatness on cardiovascular health is to do postmortem examinations on people who have died from heart attacks. If the conventional wisdom is correct, fat people should show signs of atherosclerotic damage and thin people should not. In one study of nine men who weighed at least three hundred pounds, none showed significant atherosclerosis! This sort of postmortem finding is not at all unusual.

This analysis should not be interpreted as trivializing the role of fatness in health. Clearly, given the choice, it is better not to be fat. Moreover, any sudden or large increase in weight should be brought to the attention of a doctor. What is generally forgotten is that we are not given a simple choice between being thin and being fat. There are people who have a combination of factors, which makes them very bad risks for cardiovascular health. It is a medical imperative that such people be correctly identified and given whatever help possible. However, fatness by itself is only a minor element in a complex health equation. If you are fat and free from the other risk factors, there is no reason to look upon your fat as a dangerous blight. This is particularly true if you are at or beyond middle age. This is perhaps fortunate, since, as I will show in later chapters, there is surprisingly little one can do about being fat. Unfortunately, genuine zealots along with commercial hustlers have presented fatness as *the* major health plague of our times.

Fatness is not the overwhelming medical problem it is portrayed to be. The prevalent condemnation of fat is based on a gross misinterpretation of the available data. Alas, misinterpretations of these data have become institutionalized. It bears repeating that these criticisms by no means deny that fat is a genuine health hazard under some circumstances. However, the overall importance of fat for health has been seriously overstated. The continuing confusion about when fat indicates a pathology and should be treated as opposed to when it is a benign event is itself a health hazard. The fat industry has been waging an unsuccessful war on an unfortunately intractable problem. Its efforts could be more profitably spent improving more important and more remediable deficiencies, such as smoking, improper diet, inadequate exercise, and hypertension.

If the nonexistent profat lobby were to adopt the same shoddy tactics as the antifat lobby, they could argue that thinness is dangerous and fatness is healthy. Thin or even normal weight people could find themselves listed as bad insurance risks. The profat people could cite statistics such as those presented above and still more. For example, one reputable study found that the mortality from all causes was less in fat women than in slim women. Among the Pima Indians of Arizona, the lowest mortality among males is found in men who are, by most standards, at least 50 percent overweight.

One of the rather curious statistics buried in the mountains of life insurance data is that being either very short or very tall is associated with reduced life expectancy. Yet, no one is likely to say that being short or tall causes early death. It seems more likely that any health problems in these people are related to the same exceptional physiology that caused the unusual height. Recognizing this lack of a causal relation between height and ill health suggests that even if you could do something about the height, it would not be likely to have any effect on the health problem. There are increasingly good reasons to believe that the relation between fatness and ill health may not be all that different from the height-health associations just described. Eliminating fatness would likely benefit only a small segment of the population. Unfortunately, this small segment is probably the most resistant to weight loss.

Diabetes

The relationship between diabetes and fatness is far clearer than that between heart disease and fatness. Fatness makes diabetes worse, and losing weight makes diabetes better. Few people would seriously dispute this.

Diabetes involves a functional lack of the hormone insulin. This functional deficiency can result either from not having enough insulin or from being insensitive to it. Insulin deficiency leads to elevated blood glucose levels. In diabetics, glucose is not properly used, so it accumulates in the blood. Chronically elevated blood glucose contributes to atherosclerosis. Through quite independent and poorly understood processes, diabetes also leads to damage of the small blood vessels. This latter form of vascular damage initially leads to impaired circulation and a variety of annoying problems. However, as the circulation becomes progressively worse, it causes large-scale tissue death. If this degenerative process is not arrested, it can be fatal.

Insulin is also a promoter of fat accumulation. The glucose-utilizing function of insulin is impaired in diabetics, but the fat-promoting function is unimpaired. Consequently, a vicious circle develops. In an attempt to lower blood glucose levels, the pancreas secretes more insulin. Unfortunately, the diabetic uses most of this insulin to produce fat. As the diabetic becomes fatter, his or her insulin resistance further increases and this further exacerbates the problem. Sometimes this process stabilizes at tolerable levels of blood glucose and body fat. In other cases the pancreas cannot produce enough insulin to maintain blood glucose within safe limits. In these cases the patient's life becomes dependent on insulin injections. Part of the price diabetics pay to keep their blood glucose levels down is a strong tendency to get fat.

While there is little indication that fatness causes diabetes, in someone who has a family history of diabetes fatness may precipitate the disease. On the other hand, even though fatness does not cause diabetes, weight reduction is of great benefit to diabetics. As weight is lost, the insulin resistance of the diabetic drops and the vicious circle of fat accumulation stops.

Many diabetics could get along without medication simply by losing weight. Alas, at this point a significant catch appears. Diabetics usually have even more difficulty losing weight than do nondiabetics. It's all very well to point the accusing finger and cry for austerity, privation, and health, but translating this into effective action is extremely difficult. This key issue of the efficacy of dieting will be considered in detail in chapter 5.

There is another therapeutic course open to diabetics. Insulin resistance may be dramatically improved by exercise. This improvement does not require any weight loss. This is just as well, since exercise turns out to be not a very good way to lose weight (chapter 6). Exercise is a real alternative for many fat diabetics who cannot lose weight. Alas, many fat people are so petrified by their own fat and discouraged by their inability to shed it that they often ignore readily available help. This absurd overemphasis on weight makes many of these people ignore any treatment that doesn't promise and produce weight loss. Of course, many treatments promise weight loss, but none reliably produces it.

Whereas exercise improves insulin resistance, stress appears to have the opposite effect. The stress hormone, adrenaline, is a potent insulin antagonist. For this reason, stress is particularly harmful to diabetics. However, fat diabetics in particular and fat people in general are placed under almost constant stress about their weight. They are told continually that their fat is killing them. If that isn't stressful, then nothing is. Further, diabetics soon learn that there is little they can do about their fat, and that is doubly stressful. The stress caused by an irrational fear of fat is much more harmful than the fat itself.

ARTHRITIS

Although the antifat lobbyists frequently maintain that fatness causes arthritis (and almost every other disease too), the evidence they use to support their claim is rather pathetic. The logic is that the joints of fat people are chronically overburdened and that this causes arthritis. As is so often the case, superficially this argument seems reasonable. A closer look leads to a different conclusion, however.

Curiously, it is only women who are visited with increased incidence of arthritis as a penalty for their fatness. Why men should be spared is a puzzle. This curiosity is only a minor hitch compared with the fact that fat, arthritic women do not suffer particularly in their weight-bearing joints, such as the hips and ankles. Fat women are just as likely to have arthritis of the hands! Unless these arthritic women have done a lot of rope climbing or acrobatics, their hands should not be overburdened.

A more likely explanation for the association between arthritis and fatness is that the pain of the arthritis limits activity. The limitation of activity would increase any tendency to gain weight, and the weight gain would make the arthritis more painful. This is a familiar and vicious circle. Arthritis is yet another case where fatness may exacerbate or complicate an ongoing disease without actually causing it. It is also quite possible that arthritis and fatness could be independent symptoms of something else entirely. People who are physiologically exceptional in one respect (say, fatness) are likely to be exceptional in others as well (say, arthritis).

Dieting Is a Health Hazard

This is not at all a facetious statement. The thoroughly misguided and irrational attitude toward fat and health has created a health hazard. It is little wonder that there is such widespread cynicism about even legitimate health practices.

There is another, generally ignored, reason why the people in the fat business maintain their outdated views. These people are in a business that is largely dependent on the public's unwavering belief that fat is unhealthy. Removing that prop would be very bad for business. Even apparently detached observers from the ivory tower usually have a vested interest. The vested interest of academics and scientists is research funds. The realities of research funding are such that any project that has relevance to public health problems has an improved chance of being funded. Consequently, even the most esoteric research into basic physiology and biochemistry that has any remote association with body weight is often hung on the "fat is a health menace" peg. Scientists have to stay in business, too.

As yet there isn't much of a profat business. This book is an attempt to destigmatize fat and place it in perspective. It is not meant to extol the virtues of fat or to encourage anyone to gain weight. Fat has no more inherent virtues than hair or skin, nor does it have any more inherent vices. However, if a fat lobby should develop and the merchants and hawkers set up their tents, look out. Until some enterprising individual finds the commercial alchemy that will turn fat into gold, there is not much chance of a real profat business developing. Nobody gets rich by crying, "The sky is not falling." That is just what I'm trying to tell you: The sky is not falling.

In this chapter I have tried to develop the argument that fat is a legitimate health concern for only the following main groups:

- The grossly obese (that is, if 50 percent or more of your body weight is fat)
- Those who already have signs of hypertension, heart

disease, hyperlipidemia, or diabetes, or who have a family history of any of these diseases

It should be apparent that the endangered category includes only a small proportion of the population. On the other hand, we are continually deluged with warnings that the great majority of the Western world is too fat for its own good. These scare tactics have not helped to arrest the spread of fat. People are even fatter now than before the warnings reached epidemic proportions. The scare tactics have only worked to create an atmosphere of fear about our own bodies.

Nearly everyone agrees that stress is a major health hazard. The toll exacted is difficult to quantify, but it is undoubtedly large. Fear of fat, along with a relentless and losing struggle against our own bodies would certainly rank among the top few stressors in contemporary Western society. Millions are told to lose weight when they have no need to. This would not be nearly so bad if their purgative attempts had any success, but they do not.

Weight-reducing diets do not work. Unfortunately, the more you need to lose weight, the less likely you are to be able to lose it. I'll deal with this bitter pill at length later (see chapter 5), but for the moment you'll just have to take my word for it. Since successful dieting is held to be a matter of willpower, failed dieters are held to be weak. Further, since fatness is held to be due to gluttony and sloth in the first place, failed dieters are seen as being thoroughly vice ridden. It is noteworthy that people who fail at trying to gain weight bear no such stigma. Nor are there any vices of the chronically thin that are the opposite of gluttony and sloth. Terms such as *abstemious* and *hyperactive* are generally defined as virtues.

If you are fat, you are likely to stay fat. This hard but inescapable truth does not, however, condemn you to a life of ill health. It is a great pity that because of the emphasis on fat as the root of all health woes, many fat people abandon all hope of ever being healthy. As a consequence of this, fat people often neglect all sorts of other aspects of a healthy life-style. For example, there is an emerging consensus that most people eat too much animal fat and sugar and maybe even too much protein.

At the same time, it seems that most people do not eat enough complex carbohydrates and dietary fiber.

In their despair, fat people often throw nutritional caution to the winds and immerse themselves in all the "wrong" foods. They feel that since they are condemned to being fat and unhealthy, they might at least enjoy themselves during their brief and blighted span on this earth. In their ignorance and unhappiness, they often noticeably increase their blight. These same people could undoubtedly improve both the quantity and the quality of their lives by adopting a few sensible dietary measures.

For the present argument, food may be seen as having three main components:

- Energy (measured in calories)
- Macronutrients (fats, carbohydrates, and proteins)
- Micronutrients (vitamins and minerals)

The obsession with fat has led to an almost exclusive emphasis on the energy value of food. The importance of macronutrients, in particular, continues to be neglected. Years of intensive research have done nothing to improve anyone's chances of losing weight through counting calories. At the same time, real progress has been made in the field of nutrition, particularly with respect to the importance of the macronutrient composition of the diet. As long as people are busy counting calories, they are unlikely to do much about their macronutrient intake. The antifat lobby inadvertently encourages just this sort of unhealthy nutritional practice. As long as the measure of the success of any therapeutic intervention is weight loss, the beneficial effects of sound nutritional practices will be largely ignored.

The macronutrient composition of one's diet may well be a significant factor. This most plausible effect has not been systematically investigated. It is easier to maintain a high weight if you eat a lot of fats and sugars. Fats and sugars have a much greater energy content than other foodstuffs. Fat people could well have an increased health liability because of their unhealthy diet and not simply because they are fat. The impressive cardiovascular health of fat men who live around the Mediterranean suggests that a diet low in saturated fat and high in complex carbohydrates may have protective effects. In other words, health status is not simply a function of being fat or thin. The antifat crusaders have placed an almost exclusive emphasis on the energy content of the diet while largely ignoring its macronutrient composition. This is yet another example of how fatophobia may be obscuring important health issues.

Some fat people exercise to lose weight. Sadly, exercise is no more effective in weight reduction than dieting is (see chapter 6). Unfortunately, fat people are less likely to exercise because they tend to be ridiculed, if only by silent comparison, with the Jane Fonda/Sylvester Stallone clones that stake out most exercise venues. A few raised eyebrows can do nasty things to a fat person's fragile sense of self-esteem. Although few people really overtly guffaw at fatties anymore, antifatism raises its ugly head in many more subtle, but equally destructive ways.

Most fat people do not exercise nearly as much as would be in their best interest. As is the case with the macronutrient composition of the diet, the obsessional emphasis on fat acts to drive fat people away from yet another aspect of a healthy lifestyle. Most fat people cannot lose weight, but they can substantially improve their health by exercise. Even diabetics can often greatly improve their insulin resistance simply by exercise. This improvement takes place quite apart from any weight loss.

As long as the absurd overemphasis on the importance of weight remains, millions of people will continue to be much less healthy than they could easily be. While it's true that permanently reducing weight is next to impossible for most people, improving health through exercise and sound nutritional practices are very real possibilities. Exploring these possibilities is made far less likely by current attitudes toward fatness.

The overemphasis of fatness as the source of so many health woes has had another, largely ignored adverse effect on health. It is so widely assumed that fat people are unhealthy, it is almost forgotten that there are many very healthy fat people. It is crucially important to find out how these people differ from their unhealthy compatriots. As yet, there has been almost no investigation along this line. There appears to be far more concern with associating fatness with ill health than with exploring the reasons why some fat people are so healthy. This is a particularly important area of investigation, since time after time it has been shown that weight loss is not a generally attainable goal. This highlights the importance of any other factors that can improve their health status.

An equally unhealthy consequence of the antifat hysteria is that, in their desperation, many fat people grasp at any straw that offers them hope of losing weight. Some of these straws are relatively harmless, but others are extremely dangerous. One of the most frequently grasped straws is cigarette smoking. There is a convincing body of data showing that cigarette smoking lowers body weight. Further, when smokers quit, they normally gain weight.

The weight loss produced by smoking makes taking up smoking attractive for fat people. The weight gain produced by stopping smoking compounds the difficulty in quitting. The fact that millions of people either take up or maintain smoking because of their concern about their weight is a good measure of the desperate lengths to which we have driven people. There is no longer much legitimate doubt as to the health toll exacted by smoking. Yet, in spite of the overwhelming evidence that smoking is a health hazard, many fat people choose it as the lesser of two evils.

An interesting sidelight of the smoking issue is that most smokers see cigarettes as an appetite suppressant, as well as an alternative source of oral gratification. These facts seem to support the belief that smokers weigh less because they eat less. But although cigarette smoking may be a path to weight loss (and to cancer, heart disease, emphysema, and strokes), it is probably not through reducing appetite and food intake.

Cigarettes might be expected to reduce appetite and food intake, if only because they dull the sense of taste. Surprisingly, experiments suggest that smokers eat more, not less than nonsmokers! The fact that smokers eat more, yet weigh less, indicates that smoking increases energy expenditure (see chapter 4). These findings also serve to illustrate one of the major points of this book, that how much we eat has relatively little to do with how much we weigh.

The final way in which dieting is a health hazard is that it is dependent upon and in turn supports a quite astonishing array of quackery (see chapters 5, 7, and 8). Some people might wonder what harm there is in a little idle quackery? Fat quackery is far from idle—it is one of the major health hazards of our times. This quackery continues to undermine all sorts of legitimate efforts to improve public health. A little stigma goes a long way.

CHAPTER 3

WHY ARE YOU FAT?

The belief that fatness is due to overeating and/or inactivity (gluttony and sloth) is almost as universally subscribed to as the law of gravity, but in spite of this, it is simply not true. It *is* true that fatness indicates energy intake is greater than energy expenditure. You cannot beat the laws of thermodynamics. So, in this sense, fatties must overeat and/or underexercise.

OVEREATING

When the question of whether fat people eat more than nonfat people is asked, a very different picture develops, and the real truth appears. The reasons why this most important question does not have a definitive answer is that it is nearly impossible to measure human food intake with enough precision to use it to examine the cause of differences in body weight. Even the most accurate measures of normal human food intake under controlled experimental conditions have at least a 10 percent margin of error built in. Over the period of only a year this 10 percent could result in a very large increase (approximately 20 percent) in body weight! When you remember that most people are concerned about far smaller weight gains that have appeared over much longer time spans, the inadequacy of food intake measures becomes apparent. They are not nearly precise enough to be able to pinpoint excess food intake as a cause of fatness.

One way around this difficulty is to put people on a uniform liquid diet, such as milk. With milk there is little spillage, the leftovers are easy to measure, and the energy content is very uniform. Further, milk is a reasonably complete and inexpensive diet. The problem with all liquid diets, though, is that they lack one of the most essential ingredients of the normal human diet—variety (see "Gastronomy," below).

As a result of culinary boredom, food intake on a liquid diet (or any other monotonous diet) probably bears no resemblance to a person's normal intake. The nutritionist who is trying to determine the relation between food intake and body weight is faced with an unpalatable choice. Either give people a liquid diet that is easy to measure but is likely to produce abnormal intake, or give them their normal diet and live with considerable uncertainty as to what their energy intake really is.

In fact, when one examines large groups in the population, the errors in measuring food intake become much greater than a mere 10 percent. In these large-scale-population studies, food intake is usually estimated on the basis of questionnaires or interviews. Unfortunately, we are very poor reporters of our own food intake, even when we are being totally honest. Do you really have any idea as to whether that bowl of cereal you had for breakfast weighed 25 or 75 grams?

Particularly if you are a bit fat and feel guilty about it (as almost all fat people do), or if you are concerned about your weight (as almost all lean people are), you are not likely to be an accurate recorder of your own food intake. Nor are you likely to give an interviewer very accurate information. Perhaps the one saving grace of this type of data is that whatever errors they have are just as likely to afflict group A as group B. As a result, these data are sometimes useful for comparing different groups, although they are pretty useless for pinpointing the source of fatness in any one group.

Even if you precisely weighed the individual items in each meal, the net result would not be much more useful. In a typical meal the various ingredients become so mixed up that by the end of the meal, measuring the leftover mashed potato as distinct from the peas, gravy, and butter is not possible. Further, even if you were diligent enough to try this, a fair amount of residual grease, and so forth, usually remains on the plate, on the cutlery, and on your clothes. Since this residual food matter is often particularly energy dense, the error is by no means trivial. Clearly, estimates of the net weight of food eaten under normal conditions are very imprecise.

As if this drawback were not enough, consider the next problem of converting these poor data on food intake weights into energy intakes (joules or calories). Obviously, there is a world of energetic difference between eating 100 grams of lettuce and 100 grams of chocolate. The weight of food eaten is not nearly as important as its energy value. Although it is a simple matter to obtain the energy values of most foods from the innumerable calorie counters available, these figures are also extremely imprecise. They give typical values, whereas what you actually eat may differ widely.

Identical weight samples of relatively simple foods such as fruits and meats commonly differ in their energy value by 20 to 30 percent. The energy value of more complex foods, such as salads, stews, and casseroles, is far more difficult to estimate. The only way to determine their energy value accurately is by burning a sample in a bomb calorimeter. This, of course, can only be done in a laboratory. The net result of these multiple sources of uncertainty is that under most conditions it is impossible to tell whether fat people eat more, less, or the same as nonfat people. Consequently, the assumption that people are fat because they overeat is just that, an assumption. It is supported by no data, yet nearly everyone believes it.

To further indicate just how baseless a prejudice the notion of the fat glutton is, most of the available data (inadequate as they are) show that fat people eat less than thin people! For example, a study of middle-aged men in the Netherlands showed that the fattest men tended to eat about 20 to 25 percent less than the thinnest men in the sample. In Scotland, over the period from 1964 to 1971, adolescent boys decreased their food intake by about 7 percent, yet their body fat increased by about 13 percent.

There are also a few laboratory investigations that shed some light on the relation between food intake and body weight. In one such study, over a period of thirteen days, two students whose body weights differed by only 16 percent showed a 50 percent difference in food intake. Once again, it appears that how much you eat has surprisingly little to do with how fat you are. Some people can eat twice as much as others who weigh the same.

One of the more intriguing pieces of evidence on this issue comes from an analysis of the food intake of entire nations. Interestingly, it may be easier to measure national food intake than the food intake of individuals or smaller groups. The reason for this is that there are fairly accurate data on food production as well as imports and exports of food. If you know total national food consumption in successive measuring periods, simply dividing this by population will give you a reasonable measure of changes in per capita food intake. Wastage and spillage may not be very important since they should be about the same over the successive measuring periods.

The data on national changes in food intake are surprising. For example, in Britain, as in most developed countries, total national food intake appears to have been on a slow but steady decline for two decades or more. During this same period, average body weight has been steadily increasing! These data show, yet again, that food intake is not a very good predictor of body weight. They also tend to support the view that fat people do not necessarily overeat.

Other data that should comfort the afflicted and afflict the comforted concern the role of eating "bad" foods and eating between meals. Among the first advice given to any aspiring weight loser is the injunction to avoid sweets and between-meal snacks. These are cardinal sins for the weight-conscious and are held to be bad medicine by just about everyone.

Overall food intake has been decreasing steadily over several decades in many Western countries. At the same time, the populations in these countries have been getting steadily fatter and have been eating more junk food. This suggests that the bulging of the developed nations is not simply due to eating more. It may instead be due to eating too much "sin" food, such as candies, desserts, and fast foods.

As appealing as this logic is, there are other data that fail to support it. In studies of both English workers and Israeli teenagers, those who reported themselves as eating the most of the "bad" foods were the thinnest! Similarly, the thinnest people said that they ate more meals and snacks per day than the others. These data are only self-reports, but they are nevertheless suggestive. This same issue has been approached rather more directly in military recruits who underwent a thorough dental examination at the time of their induction. The group with the most dental cavities (who presumably ate more sin food than the others) was thinner than the rest!

As with so many diet myths, the fable that fat people overeat is not just a harmless piece of folk fiction. Fat people are no more likely to overeat than are lean people, yet fat people are widely assumed to be gluttons. Eating for them, and for many nonfat people as well, is considered to be a vicious, self-destructive weakness. Millions of the afflicted carry on their foul practice (eating) covertly and reap a bitter harvest of guilt and misery.

Eating has become to the late twentieth century what masturbation was to the first part of the century. Masturbation leads to blindness and eating leads to early death. The fallacy of this is well indicated by all of us who do not require eyeglasses and by all of the old hearty eaters. Freud developed a psychology based on frustrated and misplaced sex drives as the source of psychopathology. The explosive growth of food-related psychopathology has made Freudian theory of little more than historical interest. Who will do for gastronomy what Freud did for sex?

If fatness is due to overeating, it should be possible to make thin people fat by getting them to overeat. After all, this is only what we speculate occurs to fat people in the first place. What happens when a group of volunteers overeat to gain weight? The numerous difficulties associated with precise quantification of food intake do not matter here because all you need is a more or less binary classification: one group who force themselves to eat a lot and another who carry on pretty much as normal.

One of the first of these overeating experiments was conducted on a small group of American university students. These students were encouraged to eat as much as they possibly could in order to produce a target weight gain of 20 percent. In spite of their most diligent efforts at gluttony, they typically gained less than 10 percent. Further, when their eating binge was terminated, they rapidly lost the small amount of weight they had worked so long and hard to acquire. The students clearly did not have the willpower to keep themselves fat.

The most famous of the overeating experiments was conducted on a group of prisoners in Vermont. The prisoners were set a target weight gain of approximately 15 percent. They were encouraged to achieve this end by being given unlimited and officially sanctioned access to the two cardinal vices of gluttony and sloth. Their dedication was assured by the fact that a prison doesn't provide that much in the way of alternatives.

After more than six months of strenuous overeating, many of the prisoners could not even achieve the relatively modest target of a 15 percent weight gain. This was in spite of at least doubling their food intake. Further, those who were successful in gaining weight found it very difficult to maintain their newfound fat. It seems reasonable that a 10 to 15 percent increase over their normal food intake would maintain a 10 to 15 percent increase in body weight. Surprisingly, this simple relation was not found. The prisoners found that if they did not keep up a nearly 100 percent increase in food intake, they actually began to lose weight. Imagine losing weight on a 5,000-calorie-per-day diet! One of the most successful gainers managed a 25 percent increase in weight, but had to eat 7,000 calories a day to keep his bulge. This was nearly a tripling of his normal food intake.

The above data are very important because they show that fairly modest weight gains may be exceedingly difficult to achieve and even more difficult to maintain. It seems that there is a strong physiological resistance to gaining weight. We have physiological mechanisms that defend our body weight against changes in food intake. If there was a similar physiological resistance to losing weight, it would be a nasty portent for dieting. As we will show in chapters 4 and 5, there is every indication that there is at least as much resistance to losing weight as there is to gaining it.

Resistance to losing weight may not, at first, seem to fit in with the fact that in all of these experiments the subjects rapidly lost the weight gained during the period of overfeeding. The critical difference is that when people go on slimming diets, they are usually trying to lose weight they have had for years. In contrast, in the overeating experiments the subjects were successful in reducing a weight that had been only temporarily elevated.

Having maintained the same weight for a long time makes that weight a good candidate for being "normal" even if it indicates gross obesity. Having maintained any body weight for a long time means that you have likely developed physiological mechanisms to defend it, no matter how much you may abhor it. By contrast, the Vermont prisoners still had physiological mechanisms that defended a lower weight. In this case, their physiology acted to facilitate a weight loss. In typical dieters physiological mechanisms act to inhibit weight loss.

It is interesting to compare the different manner in which permanent fatties and temporary fatties lose weight. Let us, for example, compare the response to total starvation of a 180-pound force-fed Vermont prisoner with a similar-weight prisoner who acquired his weight in the more gradual and natural manner typical of fat people. When starved, these two outwardly identical fat people would lose weight at very different rates. The "real" fat person would lose weight much more slowly than the temporary fatty. Clearly, the two fat people are not at all the same. The permanent or naturally fat person has metabolic mechanisms that inhibit weight loss. In contrast, the metabolism of the temporary or artificially fat person facilitates weight loss.

The problem with this sort of analysis is in determining just what weight a given individual will defend as a "normal" weight. Since we have physiological defense mechanisms that act to buffer our body weight against large upward or downward changes, the only real hope for losing weight lies in resetting the value of the weight we defend. Unless a readjustment of this body weight set-point takes place, any diet-induced change in body weight is likely to be both small and temporary.

Another important aspect of the Vermont experiment lies in the subjects who did not respond to the overfeeding in a typical manner. Two of the prisoners found it quite easy to gain weight, whereas the others found it to be difficult indeed. This fundamental difference shows that not everyone has similarly developed physiological defense mechanisms. Equally important is the fact that these same two prisoners had considerable difficulty losing their new weight. All of the others easily lost the weight acquired in their binge. A close examination of the medical records of the two "upwardly mobile" prisoners revealed a family history of diabetes and obesity.

A small minority of the population appears to have little difficulty gaining weight. There is probably another, even smaller minority that has little difficulty losing weight. This latter group is the dream of the diet merchants. This group may provide the few genuinely successful slimmers who appear in advertisements for weight-loss emporia and products. It is sad but true that most of the born-again slim people who appear in the ads refatten almost as quickly as they spend their appearance fees. It's only a paper moon.

As is so often the case with fatness, the closer you look, the more complex the picture becomes. Food intake may affect body weight differently depending on characteristics of the meal pattern. Animals that take all their food in one meal are far more likely to get fat than those that eat the same food as a series of snacks. In this sense, there is a distinct advantage to being a nibbler as opposed to a gorger. Nibblers are more likely to be thin, whereas gorgers are more likely to be fat.

There are probably good evolutionary reasons for this difference. Species that gorge themselves likely learned to do so because they had only occasional access to food. When you encounter food infrequently, it makes good sense to eat and store as much as possible. On the other hand, species that learned to nibble likely learned to do so because of a relatively abundant and continuous food supply. For these species, eating huge amounts and being energetically thrifty had little advantage. As a result of these evolutionary pressures, it would not be at all surprising if many species developed different ways of responding to nibbling and gorging.

There is another aspect of meal patterning that may alter the effect a given quantity of food has on your weight. It you tend to eat at night, that food energy is more likely to wind up around your waist. This is due to our being more energetically efficient at night. All of these considerations suggest that the relationship between food intake and body weight is much more complex than most people realize.

Fatness is far from a simple condition resulting from overeating. Fat people do not necessarily eat more, and how much you eat can affect your weight very differently depending on whether you are a nibbler, gorger, day eater, or night eater. Whether these findings can be put to work in a dietary context remains to be determined. Certainly, a number of wonder diets based on these principles have been major flops. As with so many diets, they succeeded at the cash register, but failed at the bathroom scales.

A superficial reading of the above section might convey the impression that food intake had nothing at all to do with body weight. That would be quite absurd. In spite of, or maybe even because of, its absurdity, this view frequently captures the imagination of the popular press. As with much of this kind of material, the motive is simply to sell newspapers. As a result, I have sometimes been cast in the role of being an advocate for untrammeled piggery. The sensation-oriented press has often portrayed these views as advocating gluttony and "damn the torpedoes" of fatness. Even worse, some have read this analysis as suggesting that gluttony is the route to slenderness. If this type of misinterpretation is not cynical and willful deceit, it is at the very least evidence of a large degree of ignorance.

The point of this section has been that food intake often does not have much to do with how much you weigh. Obviously, then, body weight is determined by other important factors besides food intake. However, it is also clear that under some circumstances changing food intake can have major effects on body weight. Fat people are not necessarily gluttons, but there are undoubtedly some fat gluttons. Once again, we are faced with the problem of separating the wheat from the chaff. This muddied issue can be clarified by examining the literature on the role of gastronomic variables in body-weight regulation in other species, such as rats and mice.

Maybe the reason that overeating is relatively ineffective in increasing body weight is that it frequently lacks the pleasurable and fundamental plus of gastronomy. Eating more of the same old boring stuff may be hard work indeed. But what about overeating when your senses are flailed and titillated by culinary delight? There is good reason to believe that these are quite different situations. Increased quantity of food eaten may have different effects than do enhancing quality and tickling the palate.

Gastronomy

Laboratory species, domestic pets, and humans rarely have difficulty regulating their weight when they eat a dreary, unvarying diet. An absolutely uniform, bland, and wholesome diet is fairly much the norm for laboratory species. This sort of diet is very rare for humans, at least in the affluent countries. The fact that laboratory species are so often kept on uniform diets whereas humans tend to be gastronomes is a major reason why laboratory data are often not nearly as relevant to the human situation as they could be. However, this lack of relevance is not due primarily to crossing any species line. It merely shows that ill-conceived experiments are not very informative. Both humans and laboratory species tend to eat a varied diet whenever they have the opportunity.

When laboratory animals or household pets are given access to rich and varied foods, the picture of the relation between food intake and body weight becomes quite different. These rich and varied diets are commonly called supermarket or cafeteria diets. Their contents cover almost every sort of culinary prohibition ever inflicted on dieters. Rats are given chocolate, peanut butter, sugared breakfast cereals, cookies, butter, and lard. The most effective diets for fattening are always very high in simple sugars and fat. Complex carbohydrates and protein are sacrificed to make the diet high in energy-dense nutrients.

Cafeteria diets often produce a large increase in food intake. If this increased intake persists for long enough, it normally results in substantial weight increases. However, after short-term cafeteria feeding, most animals rapidly lose weight as soon as they are returned to their normal diet. The weight loss is brought about by the simple expedient of voluntary undereating. It is important to note that the weight gains and the weight losses here are almost all fat. These diets have little effect on lean body mass. Cafeteria-fed rats and humans do not become bigger, they become fatter.

If the subjects are left on the cafeteria diet for a long enough period, many, but not all, appear to undergo permanent changes. When they are returned to their old, boring diet they increase their food intake in order to defend the weight gain produced by the gastronomic adventure. This suggests that prolonged gastronomy may produce an upward shift in the set-point for body weight. The parallel here with increasing fat cell number is striking. We can use dietary means to increase fat cell number and to raise the body-weight set-point. Unfortunately, we know very little about reversing the fatness or the predisposition to fatness that results from these changes.

Essentially the same pattern is found in many species, probably including humans. This sort of experiment has not been conducted as such in human beings, but there are some indications that a similar phenomenon may occur. Many groups around the world have shown large increases in fatness following prolonged exposure to "Western" diets. It may be that this is the human equivalent of the fattening of laboratory animals by exposure to cafeteria diets. As with fattened rats, if the gastronomy is carried on long enough, the fat appears to be permanent.

One of the most important observations to be made about the fatness produced by cafeteria diets is that it is a remarkably variable phenomenon. Certain strains of laboratory animals (and likely humans too) appear to be quite resistant to weight gains, even when fed the most succulent of foods. Others become junk-food addicts and blossom rapidly to formidable levels of corpulence.

Even within genetically homogeneous strains, such as albino rats, there is great variability in the susceptibility to diet-induced fatness. Littermates who are otherwise identical may show very different responses upon exposure to cafeteria diets. Because humans are far more genetically heterogeneous than laboratory species, one would expect still greater variability in their susceptibility to diet-induced fatness. At the moment we do not know how to predict who is vulnerable, nor do we know how to reverse the fatness once it is firmly established.

The message for dieters in all of this is not very cheering. Fatness looks pretty much like a one-way street. Once you've gone up it, there may be no way back. The bitterness of this pill may be softened a bit by the following consideration: If fatness were really the lethal blight that many would have us believe it is, nature would likely have given us some defense against it. The fact that, as a species, humans continue to get fatter and healthier at the same time suggests that perhaps we are not so blighted after all.

Inactivity

As we discussed above, fat people, by definition, eat more than they need. If they didn't, they couldn't be fat. However, fat people do not appear to eat more than thin people, so in this most important sense fat people do not overeat. It is quite unfair to characterize fat people as gluttons.

Attributing differences in fatness to differences in levels of physical activity is far more difficult than it may appear. The problem here is similar to that encountered with eating. Activity, like eating, is very difficult to quantify. This problem is further complicated by the fact that the same amount of movement costs more energy for fat people, because they are carrying more weight when they do it. One's overall physical condition has a lot to do with it as well. For example, the energy cost of walking for an athlete may be 60 percent less than for a nontrained person.

The increase in physical efficiency produced by athletic training should not really be surprising, since this is its aim. What is surprising is that the energy cost of sitting and even doing nothing (neither of which is as yet a recognized form of athletic pursuit) may differ greatly in people who are not athletes and are superficially identical. Relative to the whole energy economy of the organism, these differences in involuntary energy expenditure are enormous. In the period of a year these differences could make a grossly obese person return to normal weight. If the differences were in the opposite direction, they could make anyone extremely fat. These immense changes in body weight could occur even though food intake remained unchanged.

It may come as a great surprise that physical activity such as exercise only accounts for a very small proportion of our total daily energy expenditure. Perhaps the best example of this is the remarkable calculation that if a mouse were to climb the highest mountain in Great Britain, it would only increase its overall energy expenditure on that day by about 3 percent! For an average human, the same climb would produce a 22 percent increase in energy expenditure. Even this calculation may be somewhat optimistic, since after strenuous exercise most people (mice, too) typically compensate by being particularly inactive. Thus postexercise rest may partially offset the increased energy expenditure produced by exercise.

The point of this is that there is no evidence that people become fat through lack of exercise. If fat people do not eat more or exercise less, how do they become fat? The answer to this question does not really require a great deal of detective work. Fatness reflects a state of positive energy balance. When energy intake exceeds energy expenditure, the difference must be stored and our main energy storage depot is fat. The question is, how do you get to a state of positive energy balance if you do not overeat or underexercise?

We only have one form of energy intake, and that is eating. I have already explained that the answer to the cause of fatness is not there. I have also shown that the answer does not lie in activity differences. The critical point is that, in contrast to energy intake, total energy expenditure has two major components: voluntary (exercise) and involuntary. Involuntary energy expenditure (which is sometimes simply referred to as metabolic rate) normally accounts for about 80 percent of total energy expenditure. This is the obvious culprit to interrogate as to the production and maintenance of fatness.

The above analysis suggests that eating and exercise are much less important than is generally assumed in the development and maintenance of fatness. However, this criticism should not be taken to mean that the two variables are irrelevant to body weight and fatness. That would be quite incorrect. Fatness is the result of a prolonged positive energy balance, and eating and exercise are two important factors in an overall energy-balance equation.

Until the generally ignored third major element of this equation is understood, attempts to eradicate fatness will be doomed to failure. This third element is involuntary energy expenditure. A low rate of involuntary energy expenditure could explain why someone can get fat without overeating or underexercising. Conversely, a high rate of involuntary energy expenditure could explain why some people can stay thin while overeating and underexercising.

Fatness is not due simply to any one thing. Some fatness may indeed result from excessive eating and some may result from prolonged indolence. It is also likely that much of it reflects low involuntary energy expenditure. Further, these three factors interact in very complex ways. For example, eating affects energy expenditure and vice versa. The only way to reverse fatness is through prolonged negative energy balance. We will see that this simple aim is extraordinarily difficult to achieve (chapters 5 and 6).

Maybe nature is trying to tell us something. It would only be in a singularly malevolent universe that most of its earthly inhabitants would be too fat for their own good health. It seems more likely that most of the great hurrah about fatness is misplaced and unwarranted. This is just as well, since there does not appear to be much we can do about it. The sky is not falling. Chicken Little is wrong.

CHAPTER 4

THE PHYSIOLOGY OF FATNESS

There are now more than a century's worth of data showing that every significant aspect of fatness is subject to major influence by the brain. These data, which are largely from laboratory species such as the rat, nevertheless have important implications for fat humans.

The Brain

The primary involvement of the brain in regulating fatness is by no means self-evident. For a long time it was thought that body weight was regulated by a simple feedback system from the stomach. The basic idea was that the contractions of an empty stomach irritated hypothetical "hunger nerves" in the stomach wall. Eating was thought to soothe the irritated hunger nerves by distending the stomach and stopping the contractions. The fact that eating also led to an increase in body weight was seen as a rather fortunate coincidence. Alas, there is nothing that bears much resemblance to the hypothetical hunger nerve in any mammal.

On the other hand, a simple feedback mechanism like the "hunger nerve" has been shown to operate in the blowfly and is dramatically demonstrated when it is cut surgically. For when the blowfly is allowed to eat freely, it eats until it bursts. Our food intake and body weight, by contrast, are regulated by mechanisms far more complex than those in the blowfly, and that is ultimately our great good fortune.

The simple nervous system of the blowfly can be tricked all too easily. Primitive regulatory systems like that of the blowfly work well only under a very limited set of conditions. The human brain normally defends our body weight with great efficiency because of an elaborate system of checks and balances. This complexity means that it ultimately works far better and under far more conditions. The penalty we pay for our exquisite and complex energy-balance regulatory system is that it is very difficult to understand. More important, our body-weight regulatory system is very difficult to trick.

If the stomach were the critical organ that initiated eating, its removal would have easily predictable effects. If stomach contractions were the source of hunger, then removing the stomach should remove hunger. If you are not hungry, then you are not likely to eat, and if you don't eat, you should lose weight. It is essentially this sort of logic that has led to the use of various types of gastric surgery in an attempt to control gross obesity. These surgical procedures will be covered at length separately (see chapter 7). For the moment, let us confine our discussion to the effects of total stomach removal.

Stomach removal is done fairly frequently for various medical conditions quite unrelated to fatness. Total gastrectomy (stomach removal) often has surprisingly few effects on hunger. Obviously, people without a stomach cannot eat large meals, but they appear to get along quite well by eating lots of small meals. Clearly, the stomach is not essential to hunger. It was once remarked that the only reason we have a stomach is so that we may have ulcers.

The first data to show the importance of the brain in regulating body weight were provided by a nineteenth-century physician named Frölich. He had a patient who underwent a sudden and dramatic increase in both appetite and body weight. In a short period of time his weight nearly doubled. The autopsy of this patient revealed a large tumor near the base of the brain. Since the tumor had damaged both the hypothalamus and the nearby pituitary, it was not immediately clear which sort of damage caused the overeating and obesity. It took many years of careful experimentation in laboratory species to reveal that the critical region for producing these dramatic effects was the hypothalamus. The involvement of the pituitary gland was far less important.

The entire human hypothalamus is only about the size of a pea. The critical region for producing the overeating and fatness is only a small part of this tiny brain area. Damage in and around the ventromedial hypothalamic nucleus produces overeating and obesity in many species including humans. The conventional logic here is rather compelling, although, as we will show below, quite wrong. The conventional logic is that since the brain damage prevents satiety, the victim overeats.

This view depicts overeating as resulting from the inability to experience satiety. Thus, the ventromedial hypothalamic nucleus has been widely characterized as the satiety center of the brain. Inadequate satiety leads to overeating, and overeating leads to fatness. Dressed in somewhat different clothes, this same logic pervades the literature on body weight in humans without brain damage.

Before muddying this rather pretty picture, let us first make it more complete. Flanking the ventromedial hypothalamic nucleus on either side is the lateral hypothalamic area. Damage to the lateral hypothalamic area produces changes in eating and body weight that are essentially the opposite of those seen following damage to the ventromedial hypothalamic nucleus.

Lateral hypothalamic damage stops eating. The self-starvation leads to weight loss. In extreme cases this can lead to death even though food is freely available. The logic here is as follows: The brain damage prevents the experience of hunger. As a result, the victim does not eat. Because of the lack of eating, weight loss occurs. Data such as these have led to the characterization of the lateral hypothalamic area as the hunger center of the brain. Inadequate hunger leads to undereating, and undereating leads to weight loss. There, in a nutshell, is the rationale for weight-reducing diets.

Thus, hunger and satiety have been widely characterized as being centered in two adjacent parts of the brain, the lateral hypothalamic area and the ventromedial hypothalamic nucleus, respectively. The changes in weight following damage to these areas are seen as being due to changes in eating. Pick up any textbook on psychobiology, neurology, or physiology, and these concepts are sure to be there. This same "neuromythology" has been religiously carried over into the area of human nutrition. I've used the term *neuromythology* because, when it comes to the brain, the immense credibility of the public (and the scientific community, too) reaches its greatest extremes.

Dress almost anything up in neurological terms and most people will believe it. Say something is caused by a particular part of the brain and no further inquiry is needed. Unfortunately, such neurological explanations often provide answers when questions would be more appropriate. If they were real answers, it would be okay, but premature neurologizing provides pseudo answers, which all too frequently have the effect of closing further inquiry.

If our understanding of how rats regulate their weight had been reasonably extended to humans, then many of the fictions with which we are now doing battle would never have been given much credence. A common reply to this sort of cross-species analysis is, "I'm not a rat, so what does this have to do with me?" This trenchant observation can usually be met with, "You're not a bowling ball either, but you obey the law of gravity the same way the bowling ball does." Fortunately, much of the basic psychobiology of rat fatness does apply to humans.

Let us first consider the question of whether damage to the ventromedial hypothalamic nucleus really eliminates satiety. One way to approach this problem is to force-feed the animals before doing the brain damage. If the rat is fattened before the brain damage, the lack of satiety resulting from the brain damage should make it get even fatter. Instead, the evidence shows that prefattening may eliminate the voracious eating that normally follows this operation. Prefattened animals may gain little or no weight following surgery. The paradox is that in a normal animal ventromedial hypothalamic damage dramatically increases eating and body weight, whereas in a prefattened animal the same brain damage may have no effect or even reduce eating and body weight. This raises the interesting possibility that appetite and food intake may depend on body weight and not vice versa.

If the fatness that follows damage to the ventromedial hypothalamic nucleus is due to a voracious appetite, it would be instructive to put the animals on a calorie-restricted diet in order to help them recover normality. Not surprisingly, the starvation reduces their weight. However, as soon as the starved animals are allowed to eat at will, they gorge themselves and regain their former level of fatness. The parallel with human dieting is obvious.

Many experiments involving force-feeding or starvation of animals with ventromedial hypothalamic damage show that such animals can either overeat or undereat to "defend" their body weight. This defense is very much like that seen in a normal animal except that the brain-damaged animal appears to defend a weight that is far higher than in the normal animal. These animals appear to have fairly normal hunger and satiety, but they defend abnormally high body weights. These findings suggest that the ventromedial hypothalamic nucleus is not so much involved in satiety as it is in maintaining a body-weight set-point. Damage to this part of the brain raises the body weight that the organism will defend.

Conversely, it is easy to prestarve an animal before doing damage to the lateral hypothalamic area. If the brain damage eliminated hunger, prestarvation would likely have a lethal result, since the animal would be on the verge of death before the damage was inflicted. In fact, prestarved animals may actually eat vigorously immediately after the operation. The paradox is that in a normal animal, lateral hypothalamic damage eliminates eating, whereas in a starved animal the same brain damage has little or no effect on eating. Again this suggests that eating may be determined by body weight and not vice versa.

Following the lateral hypothalamic damage, it is possible to normalize the weight of the animal by force-feeding. However, after the force-feeding is stopped, the animals voluntarily starve themselves back down to their emaciated weight. Similarly, if they have not lost too much weight, it is sometimes possible to have these emaciated animals endure still further starvation. In this case, following the starvation they rapidly eat themselves back to their former level of emaciation.

As is the case with damage to the ventromedial hypothalamic nucleus, following damage to the lateral hypothalamic area the animals can either increase or decrease their food intake to defend their body weight. These data suggest that the brain damage has relatively little effect on hunger or satiety. Hypothalamic damage simply alters the weight that the animal will actively defend.

Thus it is possible to conceive of body weight as a defended physiological parameter. The set-point of the body-weight regulatory system is determined by the brain. When the set-point is challenged, the brain either initiates or terminates eating so that the weight change is minimal. According to this analysis, body weight is defended by eating or not eating just as body temperature is defended by shivering or sweating.

The implications of the set-point analysis of body weight are far-reaching. In the long term, reducing body weight by reducing eating would be about as effective as reducing body temperature by reducing shivering. Either may work in the short term, but neither is likely to be effective in the long term.

The set-point analysis is a radical and by no means universally accepted theory of body-weight regulation. One of the main things it does is to downplay the importance of eating by making eating dependent on body weight and not vice versa. Body weight may regulate eating just as body temperature regulates shivering. The traditional way of viewing the relation between eating and weight is that eating determines body weight. The set-point analysis reverses this order.

Another way the set-point analysis diminishes the importance of eating is by calling attention to the fact that body weight can change significantly even when eating remains unchanged. To illustrate this requires taking a closer look at the effects of hypothalamic damage on eating and body weight.

The fatness produced by ventromedial hypothalamic damage is usually thought to be due to overeating. Conversely, the weight loss produced by lateral hypothalamic damage is usually thought to be due to undereating. However, even if animals with ventromedial damage are prevented from overeating, they still gain weight faster than normals. Almost all of the excess weight gained is fat. The fact that fatness can occur even when eating is entirely normal is solid support for the observations that fat people are not gluttons. These findings do not mean that fat people have damage to their hypothalamus, but they do show that it is well within the realm of possibility to get fat while eating normally.

This picture is completed by a parallel set of observations on animals with lateral hypothalamic damage. In these animals the weight loss is usually thought to be due to the undereating that accompanies the brain damage. However, even if such animals are force-fed, they still tend to lose weight. These findings do not, of course, mean that slim people have brain damage, but they do show that it is possible to lose weight even when food intake is very high. Weight loss during overindulgence may be just the sort of diet the Western world is waiting for. Fortunately, not many people are so desperate that they would suffer brain damage to get thin.

There is little dispute that the brain finally organizes all of the processes that go to make someone fat, thin, or just right. Beyond this central fact, there remains a horde of important and largely unanswered questions. For example, in order to bring about the appropriate regulatory response (say eating or not eating) the brain has to get some sort of signal as to the state of your energy reserves. How does the brain know how fat you are?

Let us consider a thermostatic model of air-conditioning. In this model there is a thermometer that senses temperature. The detected temperature is then compared with the reference temperature on the thermostat. If the detected temperature is lower than the set temperature, the thermostat switches on a heater. Conversely, if the detected temperature is higher than the set temperature, the thermostat switches on a cooler. In this model there is a clear detector (the thermometer) and well-defined effectors (heater and cooler). Unfortunately, with the brain and fatness these fundamental regulatory elements are only poorly understood.

The understanding and control of fatness are impeded by the fact that we still know very little about how our brain detects fatness. For example, the fat signal cannot be visual, since blindness does not have any effect on fatness. Not only that, but many people can regulate their weight quite well without ever seeing a bathroom scale. There has even been fanciful speculation that we may have some sort of pressure sensors on the soles of our feet that produce a signal related to our weight. However, amputees and paraplegics have no special difficulty in regulating their weight.

It has become apparent that any monitoring of our body weight must be indirect. Since fat deposits do not appear to have the right sort of nerve supply to give a neural signal, it is more likely that fat is monitored by some chemical signal in the blood related to fat utilization. The nature of this signal is a subject of vigorous research.

With respect to regulating body weight or fatness, we are reaching some understanding of the nature of the effectors (these will be detailed below), but we have made much less progress in specifying the detector or, for that matter, the set-point. These deficiencies mean that it is not really clear to what extent this problem lies in the province of regulatory physiology.

As a result of the above uncertainties, much of the evidence that supports the "set-point" theory is of a somewhat indirect nature. It is, however, most important to stress that this is not just an idle academic exercise. This new approach has led to a total reanalysis of the whole issue of fat, which is in turn gradually moving this problem in new and more fruitful directions. We are hopefully putting some of the final nails in the coffin of a long and unproductive episode in the history of medicine and nutrition.

The Drive to Be Fat

For a long time fat was seen as something of a physiological accident. If you eat too much or exercise too little, you collect fat as the penalty. Fat itself is usually thought of as being the rather passive outcome of all sorts of other processes. This old view is changing. There is now a great deal of evidence that fat should be thought of as another organ with its own functions and, more importantly, with its own protective mechanisms. Much of this revolution has resulted from studies of fat-cell size and number.

Most humans have about 250 billion fat cells. Each of these fat cells typically weighs about 600 nanograms. A fast juggling of exponents comes up with a total fat weight of about 30 pounds per average person. This is exactly the total fat weight for a normal, adult male. Becoming fat involves increasing fat-cell size and/or number. This scheme allows for three quite different types of fatness. Fatness can be primarily due to increased fat-cell size, to increased fat-cell number, or to both. Interestingly, these different types of fatness appear to be different in several important respects. In other words, fat is not simply fat.

Fatness that is characterized by increased fat-cell size is called *hypertrophic,* whereas when it is characterized by increased fat-cell number it is called *hyperplastic.* There are data showing that if you have a large number of fat cells, your fatness will be more resistant to treatment than if you simply have a normal number of very full fat cells. That is, hypertrophic fatness may be easier to treat than hyperplastic fatness.

Dieting can reduce fat-cell size but not number. It has been shown that in fat people who are on severe diets, weight loss slows drastically when fat-cell size approaches normal. It appears that number of fat cells is more closely regulated than is total fat mass. The implication of this is, of course, that once you have too many fat cells, you will have a permanent tendency to be fat.

It was once thought that fat-cell number was determined genetically and/or in the very early stages of life. As a consequence, there have been a number of attempts to nip obesity in the bud by intervening in the early stages of life. The most obvious thing to do is to effect early starvation in order to prevent or reverse the proliferation of fat cells. Obviously, this cannot be done in humans, but it has been done in rats.

In genetically fat rats, early starvation reduces fat-cell size but not fat-cell number. In fact, if the starvation is severe enough, genetically fat rats will sacrifice muscle and brain before fat. Infantile starvation of these rats results in stunted, retarded rats that are still quite fat.

Many experiments such as these indicate that fat is not simply the incidental outcome of balancing other equations. Fat is not some sort of penalty we pay for not taking proper care of ourselves. Fat is, instead, a distinct entity, another organ of our body, with its own functions and protective mechanisms. The fact that a starving rat may burn up its own brain in preference to its fat attests to just how powerful the fat-defense mechanisms can be.

It has recently been shown that long-term feeding of rats on diets high in sugars and fats ("cafeteria" diets) may increase fat-cell number even in adults. These data are particularly important because it is widely believed that fat-cell numbers are fixed in childhood. This means that fat-cell numbers are more flexible than was previously thought. The problem is that while we are gaining some knowledge as to how fat-cell number may be increased, we have made little progress as to how to reduce their number. If increases in fat-cell number are really irreversible, it is bad news for aspiring weight losers.

The fat-cell data join a larger body of data that suggests some people were made to be fat. For naturally fat people, slenderizing may involve thwarting a strong biological predisposition. Even if this were possible (which is highly doubtful), they will always have a powerful physiological pressure in the direction of fatness. In cases like this, slimness may only be achieved at the price of chronic physiological and psychological stress. Any sane cost-benefit analysis of this situation would suggest that the damage produced by chronic stress is just too high a price to pay for slenderness. The exception to this is those few unfortunates who are genuinely endangered by their fat (see chapter 2).

This analysis is further complicated by the fact that it assumes that choosing slenderness is a viable choice if you are willing to pay the bill in stress. In fact, very few aspiring slimmers really have the option of choosing slenderness at any price. The great majority of slimmers pay the price in stress without even reaping the dubious benefits of weight loss. Findings such as these cast further doubts on the wisdom of indiscriminately attacking all fat. Although fat does merit a full-scale attack in some people, there are many more people whose fat should be left alone. As long as we continue to confuse genuinely malignant fatness with the far more prevalent benign fatness, it will be to the harm of everyone.

Energy Balance

At last, there is just now emerging a coherent conceptual framework for considering human fatness, and it may well create order out of the existing chaos. This concept has been around for a while, but it has taken some time to get its head above the crowd. We will try to spell out below just why fatness can be subsumed under the heading of "Energy Balance." It should become apparent that the energy-balance approach is the only way to fully understand fatness.

It will make this discussion a great deal easier for all of us if we can express the whole problem as a simple equation.

$$E_{in} = E_{out} + E_{stored}$$

Like so many simple equations, this one turns out to be very complex indeed. For the moment, however, let us admire its simplicity. What the equation means is that *Energy Intake = Energy Output + Energy Stored.* When $E_{in} = E_{out}$, no energy is stored. This represents a biological system in perfect equilibrium. Like all ideal states, a perfect equilibrium of energy processes probably never exists. However, if we could maintain this perfect state of energy balance, our weight would never change.

It has become standard practice to express E_{in} and all of the other elements of this problem in heat units, such as the j (joule) or cal (calorie). Because these are such small units, they usually appear with the prefix *kilo* (thousand) or *mega* (million). Thus the standard units of energy balance are kj, kcal, mj, and, mcal.

The reason that a truly balanced energy equation almost never occurs is that energy expenditure (E_{out}) is continuous, whereas energy intake (E_{in}) is very irregular. We eat only occasionally. Even if we are in a coma, we expend a surprisingly large amount of energy—the minimal amount of energy that is required to sustain life. This energy is used to maintain body temperature and muscle tone as well as to keep all of our other physiological machinery running. Even in a coma our brain must function; we must breathe and circulate our blood.

Living humans constantly alternate between states of positive and negative energy balance. The only time we ever achieve a long-term steady state of energy balance is when we are dead. In positive energy balance (when E_{in} is greater than E_{out}) the energy difference is stored. As mentioned earlier, excess energy is stored as fat, glucose, or glycogen. Conversely, in negative energy balance (when E_{out} is greater than E_{in}), the energy shortfall must be taken from the stores of fat, glucose, or glycogen. All energy has to come from somewhere and go somewhere. In lean times we draw on our stores and in lush times we add to our stores.

All of this looks terribly simple, but as you might have guessed, energy balance is far from simple. Although there are only three elements in the energy-balance equation (input, output, and storage), their interrelationships are rather poorly understood. Changing any one of these elements may change both of the others. Even if one element remains quite constant, the other two may vary widely. For example, given exactly the same food intake as person B, person A may lose weight, whereas person B may gain weight. Similarly, two people with widely differing food intakes may have identical weights. Numerous examples of this sort of weight/food-intake dissociation were cited above.

While energy intake and storage are relatively easy to see, energy output is far more difficult to measure. As a result, we know far less about it. Since all of the elements of the energy-balance equation have been discussed in various places above, we can now look at them in a little more depth.

E_{in} consists solely of food. Energy is obtained from the food by combining it with oxygen (O_2). This combustion process liberates energy much like the combustion of fuel in any engine. The gross energy value of any food is the heat it produces when burned. Nutritionists measure this value as the heat liberated during combustion, using a device called a bomb calorimeter. However, although almost anything can be burned in a bomb calorimeter, there are a number of food elements that humans cannot oxidize. For example, cellulose and some related plant fibers (both complex carbohydrates) burn completely in a calorimeter, but they pass through the human digestive tract pretty much intact. Sheep and cows use these same complex carbohydrates for most of their energy.

The recently-in-vogue "high-fiber" diets intentionally maximize the difference between the gross energy and the digestible energy of foods. There seems to be little doubt that many people eat diets that are too digestible for their own good health. However, as we will discuss later, adding indigestible elements to food likely has very little effect on either food intake or body weight. Unfortunately, since fiber supplements are of little use in weight reduction, many come to feel that dietary fiber is not important to health. The contagion from failure to reduce weight casts doubt on yet another valid health issue. This is just one of the ways in which the obsession with dieting is so harmful.

The digestible energy value of any food does not really indicate how much energy will be available to use and/or store. The difference results from the fact that we do not completely oxidize everything we digest. Incomplete oxidation is common with proteins. On the other hand, fats and carbohydrates are normally completely oxidized. The incompletely oxidized products of proteins in the food are excreted in the urine.

The net or useful energy in any food is the difference between its digestible energy and the energy you ultimately excrete. Fortunately, the energy-accounting processes here are somewhat simplified by the fact that in the great majority of human diets, the energy excreted is quite constant. Normally, humans excrete about 5 percent of total energy intake. As much as we might like the idea of being able to excrete a larger part of what we eat, this figure rarely changes. Even diuretics and laxatives do little more than temporarily increase water loss. The only time that we excrete much more than 5 percent of our energy intake is when we have a serious illness. A really nasty disease remains the most effective way of losing weight.

Overall, there is nothing conceptually difficult about the E_{in} part of the energy-balance equation. What is difficult about E_{in} is measuring it. Although precise day-to-day measurements of E_{in} are impossible under normal circumstances, there are accurate measures of the energy values of the major classes of macronutrients. These are presented in the table below.

NUTRIENT	ENERGY VALUE (CAL./OZ.)
Protein	140
Fat	310
Carbohydrate	130
Alcohol	240

It may come as a surprise to some that alcohol joins the trio of the major macronutrients, but unlike all other foods, alcohol is not simply a combination of proteins, fats, and carbohydrates—alcohol is alcohol. Further, alcohol is a major source of energy for many millions of people. Not only is alcohol a very rich source of energy, but 100 percent of it is used. Alcohol is also absorbed from the gastrointestinal tract more rapidly than any other substance. Although fat contains more energy than alcohol does and fat is almost as completely used, fat is absorbed much more slowly.

The most complex and probably the most important element of the energy balance equation is E_{out}. When we think of energy output, we tend to think of exercise and other forms of voluntary activity. In fact, these forms of energy expenditure are relatively minor in our whole energy economy. Even in extremely active animals, such as mountain goats, voluntary activity probably accounts for only about 5 percent of their total daily energy expenditure. The application of this figure to humans is not straightforward, since, in large animals, activity is much more energetically expensive than it is in small animals. However, even in large animals, such as humans, voluntary activity rarely counts for more than about 20 percent of total daily energy expenditure.

Since we engage in so many obligatory forms of activity such as getting dressed, walking around, and climbing stairs, additional recreational activities such as playing tennis or jogging do surprisingly little to increase overall energy expenditure. Climbing the highest mountain in Britain would only increase energy expenditure by about 20 percent. Even this relatively modest amount (it is a relatively modest mountain) could be somewhat of an overestimate, since after strenuous activity most people tend to compensate by being particularly inactive.

There are data suggesting that after strenuous exercise, energy expenditure may remain elevated. This elevation has been said to persist even when we try to compensate by being inactive. Even if this is the case, very few people have the time to significantly increase their energy expenditure by exercise. While the expression "a mountain a day keeps fatness away" may be true, very few of us could or would want to be so preoccupied with exertion. As we will discuss later, this limitation does not detract from the health value of exercise, but it does suggest that exercise is a fairly minor element in our overall energy expenditure. Thus, exercise is not likely to be a very effective way of losing weight. This issue will be discussed at some length in chapter 6.

Since voluntary activity accounts for only about 20 percent of our daily energy expenditure, there remains the problem of accounting for the other 80 percent. Here things start to get a little tricky. The obvious answer would seem to be that the remaining 80 percent goes to keeping our hearts pumping, lungs breathing, brain operating, body temperature and muscle tone maintained, and tissue repaired, not to mention growth and reproduction. But the truth is that this only applies in the case of a starving person. The reasons why this does not apply to fed people are very close to the heart of the problem of what causes fatness.

When a starving person eats, the energy obtained from the food is fully utilized in the maintenance operations described above. However, the exemplary efficiency of energy use during starvation is the exception to a more general rule of wasting energy when we are not starved. This wastage takes the form of converting food energy into heat. The heat is radiated into our surroundings. A starving person is pretty much 100 percent efficient in using available energy. In contrast, a fed person may waste a good deal of energy as radiated heat. This heat wastage is usually called diet-induced thermogenesis. So you see that there are really only three things you can do with food energy: you can use it, you can store it, or you can waste it.

In evolutionary terms, energy wastage might seem to be something of a mistake or a design error. Wouldn't it be a better idea to maximally use all of the energy at our disposal? However, on closer scrutiny energy wastage turns out to make very good sense. If we did not have some mechanism for energy wastage, our body weight would "follow" our food intake very closely. Increasing food intake would result in an increase in body weight. The problem this sort of arrangement would raise is that if the levels of any essential nutrient in our diet were reduced, we would have to eat more just to maintain minimal levels of the key nutrient. This, of course, would inevitably lead to weight gain. If the level of the nutrient were chronically low, gross obesity would result. Thermal-wastage mechanisms allow us to overeat when needed.

Like other aspects of our physiology, being able to overeat

is no longer of much adaptive value. The availability of essential nutrients rarely changes much anymore, at least in the affluent world. On the other hand, being able to overeat without paying the price of fatness can be a lot of fun. It's really quite astonishing that in the vast lore that has accumulated about fatness the word *fun* appears so infrequently. This puritanical streak is far too dominant in the weight business.

The fact that diet-induced thermogenesis is a critical mechanism in defending us against large increases in body weight leads to some obvious conclusions. Particularly efficient thermogenic mechanisms would make it very difficult to gain weight, which seems to be the case with young people. This is reflected in the well-known fact that fatness increases steadily with age. Teenagers, in particular, can often eat immense quantities without gaining much weight.

If all excess food energy is converted into heat, it is impossible to gain weight no matter how much one eats. The remarkable ability of diet-induced thermogenesis to compensate for overeating has been best demonstrated in young pigs. Growing pigs were fed an extremely low-protein diet. In order to get enough protein from this unbalanced diet they had to eat five times as much as pigs on a normal diet, but what is nearly miraculous is that they did not gain any more weight than pigs on a normal diet.

I should quickly add that in humans the lofty ideal of thermogenesis fully compensating for overeating remains an unattained ideal. It is not likely that it will ever be achieved. What is important about this finding is that it suggests that if there is a road out of the fat wilderness, it will involve increasing thermogenesis. The more thermogenic capacity you have, the less likely it is that you will become fat.

The converse of this ideal (inadequate thermogenesis) would produce a strong tendency toward becoming fat. In this sort of affliction, any energy intake that was not quickly used would be stored as fat.

There is an increasing body of evidence that suggests that at least some human fatness involves deficient thermogenesis. The situation may be succinctly described as follows. Being energy inefficient predisposes one toward slenderness. Being energy efficient predisposes one toward fatness.

The importance of thermogenesis in regulating body weight has been elegantly demonstrated in humans. Experimenters measured energy expenditure before and after a highly sugared drink. Fat subjects showed a much smaller increase in energy expenditure than did normal-weight subjects. In other words, the fat subjects retained more energy from an identical-size meal. These data suggest than lean people are protected from fatness by adaptive thermogenic responses. Conversely, some fat people may be predisposed to fatness by maladaptive thermogenic responses.

The astute reader might well raise the point that perhaps the low thermal wastage of the fat people was a result of the fatness and not its cause. This point was also addressed in the above experiments. The very lowest thermal wastage was seen in people who were formerly fat!

Together these results paint a rather convincing picture. Some people have a clear-cut metabolic bias toward fatness. It consists of a subnormal thermal wastage of food energy. The fact that this metabolic deficiency persists even after weight loss means that such people will find it particularly difficult to maintain their weight loss.

The above findings on thermal wastage also have important implications for other metabolic investigations of fat people. Numerous studies have failed to show that the resting-energy expenditure of fat people is less than that of normal-weight people. This lack of a difference has been misused. It has been used as evidence for the view that fatness is due to overeating and not to any thermogenic irregularity. These new data suggest that looking for differences in resting-energy expenditure has been barking up the wrong metabolic tree. The essential metabolic difference between fat and nonfat people may well be related to differences in diet-induced thermogenesis.

Some strains of laboratory animals are genetically fat. This genetic predisposition is not simply an expression of gluttony. Even if their food intake is forcibly held to "normal" levels, they still get fat. These animals do not just get bigger; their extra weight is almost exclusively fat. They also experience particular difficulties in maintaining their body temperature in the cold.

Normal animals can use very large amounts of energy to

maintain their body temperature in the cold. Genetically fat rats appear to lack this heat-producing ability. Genetically fat rats are good at producing fat, but they are very poor at producing heat. Clearly, their metabolism is shifted toward storage at the expense of sacrificing thermogenic ability.

If thermogenesis is so important, you would think that there would be a special thermogenic organ. In fact, there is a thermogenic organ or perhaps even group of organs. We have a special kind of fat tissue called *brown adipose tissue*, or, more simply, *brown fat*. Brown fat was first discovered in connection with investigations of adaptation to cold. The activity and perhaps even the amount of brown fat increases with exposure to cold. It was once thought that the main physiological way to produce heat was by shivering. The other means of producing heat are, of course, behavioral measures, such as seeking shelter, putting on more clothes, or lighting a fire. However, infants are not very good at putting on clothes, lighting fires, or shivering.

The ability of infants to produce a great deal of heat appears to be largely due to their brown fat. All living tissue produces heat as a consequence of doing other things, but brown fat's only function is to produce heat. Brown fat is specialized in the execution of "futile" metabolic cycles. In these cycles, A is converted to B, and then B is converted back to A. The net result of this activity is no change, hence the term *futile*. However, each of the steps uses energy and therefore produces heat.

The thermogenic ability of brown fat is very large. As little as 2 ounces of brown fat can increase human energy expenditure by nearly 25 percent. A reduction in energy expenditure of 25 percent would, over the course of a year, result in a weight gain of about 50 pounds, even if food intake did not change at all. In young rodents the thermogenic ability of brown fat is even more impressive than it is in humans. Rodent brown fat can increase overall energy expenditure by as much as 200 percent! In order to do this without itself catching fire, the brown fat must be cooled by additional blood flow.

The blood flow to brown fat may increase by as much as fifteenfold. When the demand to produce heat is maximal, rodent brown fat can receive over a third of the animal's total blood flow. The rather inferior heat-producing performance of human brown fat results from the fact that we do not have as much of it (relatively speaking) as do many other species. Nevertheless, our meager 2 ounces of brown fat has the potential to make the difference between slenderness and gross obesity.

Until quite recently it was thought that humans only had brown fat during infancy. Certainly, brown fat is more obvious in the young of all species, but there may still be substantial amounts left even in adults. It is particularly apparent in full-grown hibernating animals, such as the bear. These animals use their brown fat to elevate their body temperature when coming out of hibernation in the spring.

The pronounced decline in human brown fat occurs around the age of thirty. This is also the age at which the dreaded middle-age spread begins to appear. It is probably premature to attribute middle-age spread entirely to the decline in brown fat, but at the moment brown fat does look like a pretty good candidate.

The controversy surrounding the role of brown fat in humans is one of the most vigorous in the current literature. Besides calling attention to the importance of thermogenesis in body-weight regulation, the brown fat issue has further highlighted the importance of species differences in this area. It is now beyond dispute that brown fat is an important thermogenic organ in many species. It is rather less certain as to its importance in adult humans.

It is just possible that brown fat itself is a bit of a red herring. Brown fat has been said to be responsible for the formidable amount of thermogenesis which humans seem capable of. This may be asking too much of what is, by even the most optimistic accounts, a tiny piece of tissue. There are some very recent data showing that the maximum thermogenic capacity of the rat is far greater than that which could be produced by even the most totally turned-on brown fat. This finding suggests that there may be another thermogenic organ, which is perhaps even more important than brown fat.

The other thermogenic organ could be skeletal muscle. Besides doing its usual work of moving us around, skeletal muscle may also be capable of generating heat in the quiescent state. Even if skeletal muscle had only quite small thermogenic abilities, the fact that we have so much of it could easily make it the primary thermogenic organ. The furor surrounding brown fat may have obscured the possibility that it could be only a relatively minor factor in overall thermogenesis. This controversy by no means diminishes the importance of thermogenesis in weight regulation.

Is It Your Glands?

Fat people have been forced to assume a defensive posture for some time. One of the first officially sanctioned lines of defense for fat people was, "It's my glands." Gluttony and sloth have always been held to be voluntary vices for which the fat person is directly responsible. On the other hand, a glandular affliction usually carries with it a certain degree of absolution from the burden of sin. It is little wonder that so many fat people have sought this sort of explanation for themselves. The thyroid gland has provided a degree of exculpation rarely found outside of churches.

The readiness of fat people to blame their thyroids for all their woes is indicative of some curious prejudices. One reason that the thyroid is seen as an attractive crutch is that thyroid dysfunction is more remediable than character faults such as gluttony and sloth. There is a widespread belief that physical problems are more real, justifiable, and curable than psychological problems. If you have a thyroid problem, you are merely sick, but if you have a psychological problem, you are weak or crazy. In the case of sickness, you cannot be held responsible by the general public, but madness is a more negative reflection on the victim. These Neanderthal views are not merely wrong, they are harmful.

Thyroid hormones are involved in numerous aspects of energy utilization and expenditure. Diseases involving underactivity and overactivity of the thyroid are often respectively associated with fatness and thinness. However, there is very little indication that fat people in general have anything wrong with their thyroids. The occasional study has shown some sort of thyroid dysfunction in some fat people. This is the exception to the more general rule of fat people having pretty much normal thyroid function. Perhaps more important than these clinical data are the results of using thyroid preparations to lose weight. The dozens of commercially available thyroid potions, tonics, and elixirs are of no help in losing weight. They fatten the vendor and fleece the purchaser (see chapter 7).

The thyroid myth does serve the purpose of calling attention to the broader issue of hormonal effects on body weight. Almost all hormones can, under certain circumstances, produce changes in body weight. Further, a number of these hormones can be shown to be significantly altered in massively obese humans. Quite apart from the chicken-and-egg problem raised by these data is the fact that the hormonal status of the vast majority of fat people is quite normal. At the moment, it seems rather unlikely that hormones and the endocrine system hold the keys to fatness.

CHAPTER 5

FIGHTING FAT WITH DIETS

In the final analysis, cautioning people that their fat may not be so unhealthy often has little effect. Convincing them that their fat is not ugly is a still more difficult task. Trying to destigmatize fat and place it in its proper perspective often does little to stem the tide, which has been running for many years.

Diet Madness

For better or worse, a very large number of people want to lose weight. Many of these aspirants to slenderness are not even sure why they want to be thinner. They express their yearning in vague terms, such as "I just feel better when I'm lighter." Expressions of this sort are usually a reflection of the pervasive antifat feelings in the community. These people may in fact feel better when they are not fat, but it is probably due more to a relief from social stigma than to a loss of weight.

It is sad to think that many women who want to lose weight are not really fat but believe themselves to be. These women are the victims of an irrational fatophobia, which has radically elevated the status of emaciation. Traditionally, thinness was seen as a harbinger of death that must be avoided at all costs. Now, in many circles, thinness is seen as a cardinal virtue that must be attained at any cost. How much do you want to bend your physiology in order to fit in with this year's model of the ideal woman? It turns out that even if you really don't mind attacking your own physiology, there is probably not much you can do other than injure your health and self-esteem.

Sooner or later the majority of adults in Western societies try a weight-reducing diet. The rationale for these diets is always pretty much the same. Fatness comes from overeating, hence slenderness will follow undereating. Diets are dressed in all sorts of different costumes, but underneath the wrapping they usually vary only in minor details. There are solid, conservative diets based upon sound physiological principles. There are the crazy, fad diets based upon an ageless amalgam of ignorance and greed. All of this exists in the face of increasing evidence that fatness is not necessarily due to overeating and that undereating does not necessarily lead to slenderness.

The pervasiveness of the fear and loathing of fat is extraordinary. It is no longer an exceptional feeling, it is rather the norm in many segments of society. A recent survey of schoolgirls in San Francisco revealed some shocking statistics. Nearly half of the nine-year-olds questioned were dieting! Of the seventeen-year-olds, nearly 90 percent were dieting. In this group approximately 60 percent thought they were overweight, while the researchers found that less than 20 percent of them were actually overweight. This means that about 70 percent of the young girls were subjecting themselves to needless privation. Worse, many of the more radical diets may cause serious and long-term physiological and psychological damage. In addition, many have risked their lives through the abuse of laxatives and various diet pills. Diet-related deaths constitute a very significant source of mortality in young people. This is ugly, sad, and needless.

Ultimately, the establishment and the lunatic fringe are united by their common failure to change fatness into slenderness. The continuous proliferation of diets is adequate testimony to their failure. If any diet were as successful as its proponents claim, the entire world would know about it in a matter of days. There would be only that one universal diet and worldwide rejoicing. Needless to say, this fairy-tale scenario has not taken place, nor is it likely to. The uniform failure of diets, sensible or otherwise, has generated a bewildering array of "alternative" treatments for fatness (see chapter 7). Fatness has its own alchemy.

Alchemy, like the fear of fat itself is a product of ignorance and impotence. There is an enormous pressure to be slim and beautiful. This is further compounded by medical advice advocating slenderness as the road to good health. One of the most common health prescriptions of our times is the common parting advice of the physician: "And it wouldn't hurt to lose a little weight, either." Alas, physicians are little better at bringing about weight loss than the commercial hustlers and quacks.

There is an important difference between the ineffective treatments of the medical profession and those of the commercial hustlers. Medical advice is much less likely to be overtly harmful. Almost any physician is much better equipped to look after your health than almost any nonphysician. In addition, although the efforts of physicians in this regard are often naive or ill advised, their intentions are usually impeccable. They may be fools, but they are rarely knaves. This is not always the case with entrepreneurs. Often their sole interest in your fat is in turning it into a profit. Knaves abound in this area, but few of them will have M.D. after their name.

What matters about a diet is not its logic or who pushes it or their motives. There are only two questions you need to ask about any diet. One is, does it work? The other is, what does it cost? The cost is not merely to be measured in terms of money, but in terms of the health and happiness of the dieter. A conspicuous feature of the rare cases of successful dieting is the high price they pay for slenderness.

Most successful dieters lead lives of continual privation centered around an obsessional preoccupation with their weight. Many develop serious eating disorders, such as anorexia nervosa or bulimia (see chapter 8). It appears that very few are really happy. Almost nobody bothers to ask these rare successes if their lives have been improved by losing weight. The typical successful dieter is characterized by a grim resignation and not a little bitterness. These and other considerations suggest that there is often real reason to doubt whether successful dieters are better off than failed dieters.

The purpose of a diet is to lose fat, not just to lose weight. This essential fact is sometimes lost in the desperate struggle to lose weight. It is just this kind of desperation that drives people to abuse laxatives and diuretics. It is this same desperation that brings tears of joy to dieters' eyes when they weigh themselves after two or three days on a diet. Laxatives, diuretics, and a few days of dieting merely cause a transient loss of water. They do not touch your fat.

In order to lose fat, energy intake must be less than energy expenditure. This state of negative energy balance must be maintained for a substantial period of time. Weight loss absolutely requires negative energy balance. Dieters cannot beat the energy-balance equation any more than high jumpers can beat the law of gravity.

The illogic of the diet charlatans is epitomized by statements like "Eat fat and grow slim" and "Calories don't count." It is a curiosity of human nature that when levitationists are debunked, their demise is by no means assured. The same obtains with diet gurus. When their products are shown to be silly or even harmful, few of their customers heed the warnings. It would seem that many people do not want to know the truth. It is also obvious that there is big money in diet hoaxes. A lot of people are very frightened.

In the relatively rare cases when diet gurus are debunked, the cold, hard facts usually do not filter far beyond the walls of academia. The market for flamboyant stupidity seems boundless. Often the very fact that their nonsense is attacked by the establishment is perverted by the diet gurus into evidence of the real value of their snake medicine. Medical criticism is often welcomed by these people as a sign of recognition. It is as close to legitimacy as most of them will ever get.

Frequently, the diet gurus are elevated to the status of international celebrities. The more bizarre the new wonder weight-loss plan, the more prostrate the public becomes at the guru's feet. Words like *amazing, incredible,* and *unbelievable* abound. Obviously the public is rather more credulous (and much more desperate) about fat than it is about gravity.

The following section is an analysis of the logic behind and practice of some of the major contemporary diet trends. It is by no means comprehensive, since diets proliferate so quickly that by the time this book hits the streets, there will be dozens of new schemes on the market. Fortunately, the present arguments will not be at all out of date. On the contrary, the "amazing" and "new" diets that appear weekly are invariably just slight twists or shallow repackaging of a relatively small number of core themes. It is these major themes that will be explored below.

Low-Energy Diets

Shedding fat requires the use of our energy reserves. This can only be done by making energy intake less than energy expenditure. This is a simple, markedly nonmagical concept. Consequently, at the very outset of this section it should be noted that the only diets that have any validity at all are low-energy diets. If any other diet has any genuine effect, it can ultimately only be through producing negative energy balance.

One problem with shedding fat by restricting energy intake is that fat is such a good source of energy. Consequently, it takes a lot of energy-intake restriction to use up relatively little fat. A little fat goes a long way. Fat evolved for this very reason. The energy value of fat is about 5,000 kcal per pound. Since a typical adult diet has about 2,600 kcal per day, it is easy to calculate how much dieting you have to do to shed a given amount of fat. It takes nearly two days of total starvation to use one pound of fat. Diets that are less than starvation take correspondingly more time to use up fat.

A 40 percent reduction in energy intake would save about 1,000 kcal per day. This figure makes the optimistic assumption that there is no compensatory reduction in energy expenditure. Since the energy value of fat is 5,000 kcal per pound this sort of diet would take over four days to shed one pound of fat. Along the way you might well lose several pounds of water (see below), but this is only apparent, not real weight loss.

More severe diets produce more rapid weight losses, but it is still a very slow procedure. Even a fairly radical diet of 800 kcal per day requires over two days to use one pound of fat. Remember that these figures are based on the assumption that there is no reduction in energy expenditure in response to the diet. Particularly in very fat people and in diets of longer duration, energy expenditure may decrease so that the use of one pound of fat may well take as much as four days even on a very severe diet.

The high energy density of fat, along with the reduction in energy expenditure that occurs during dieting, makes the dieter's task formidable indeed. The rapid loss of four to five pounds at the start of most diets, merely reflects the loss of water resulting from using glycogen. This is not true weight loss in the sense of shedding fat. The weight loss at the beginning of diets is merely a transient drying up. If you can get genuinely enthusiastic about this sort of weight loss, you are probably the type who spits before weighing yourself.

At about the same time that a diet depletes the small stores of glycogen in the liver and muscles, your body gets the message that you are starving. Alas, the body does not seem to appreciate our efforts to sculpt it into a more elegant shape. The body blindly responds to dieting in the same manner it responds to any form of starvation. The body's age-old response to starvation is to become energetically efficient. The wasteful loss of heat that normally follows eating (diet-induced thermogenesis) is eliminated within a few days of the start of most diets. When your body starts to metabolically fight weight loss, the hard part of the diet has just begun.

When metabolic compensation occurs, the initial weight loss begins to diminish or even reverse. It is at this point that most dieters become discouraged and give up. As millions can testify, it is entirely possible to lose no weight at all after a few days on 1,000 kcal/day. This 60 percent reduction from normal food intake is extremely stressful and unpleasant for many people, yet in many cases it is not enough to produce more than a small and transient weight loss.

Substantial weight loss usually requires an energy intake of about 750 kcal/day. Even on a radical diet such as this, weight loss declines sharply after a week or so. It is at this critical point that counseling can be of benefit. If dieters are told that their rate of weight loss will decrease appreciably, some of the disappointment may be avoided. This by itself can lower the very high early drop-out rate from diets. Whether such counseling has any beneficial long-term effects is more doubtful.

It may come as a relief to many that the ability of the body to compensate for reduced energy intake is finite. We can only reduce our energy wastage so much and then fat must be used to provide the energy that would normally come from current food intake. Energy has to come from somewhere. If it does not come from our current intake, it must come from our stores.

Unfortunately, many dieters (particularly very fat ones) show a great reluctance to get into their fat deposits. Even though all of their short-term reserves (glucose and glycogen) are exhausted, many such people spare their fat. Their only alternative is to use appreciable amounts of muscle protein. The premature use of muscle protein for energy is only one of the factors responsible for the unusual weakness and fatigue that many dieters suffer.

One way that diet gurus deal with the destructive loss of muscle protein that occurs during diets is to ignore it. This is quite easy, since most diet gurus have only very vague and confused ideas as to what physiological changes take place during diets. Their primary interests are commercial, not physiological. Another approach is to tackle the problem head-on and design a diet that is "protein sparing." The ideal of a protein-sparing diet is extremely difficult to achieve. One of the most publicized attempts in this direction (see "Liquid-Protein Diets," below) is also one of the most dangerous diets ever foisted upon a gullible public.

Let us say that you use this book to thread your way through the maze of silly diets and have come up with one that is sensible. A sensible diet reduces energy intake and provides a reasonable level of basic nutrients. Surprisingly, there are lots of sensible diets around, but they tend to be obscured by the fad and lunatic fringe diets, which breed like flies. Let us further say that you really are determined to lose weight, so you supplement your diet with a program of regular exercise.

At numerous points in this book you will have undoubtedly got the message that I am very skeptical about diets and exercise (see chapter 6) as instruments of weight loss. Dieting and exercise certainly do not guarantee weight loss, but on the other hand, they do make weight loss more likely than if you do nothing at all. By the same token, gluttony and sloth do not guarantee fatness, but they do make it more likely. So you can maximize the likelihood of your losing weight by a good diet and sound exercise.

Following this commonsense prescription gives you about as good a chance as you can have of losing weight. Unfortunately, even with this maximizing strategy, less than 10 percent of dieters ever lose anything approaching their target weight loss.

The 10 percent who do lose substantial amounts of weight are testimony that real weight loss is possible. the 90 percent who fail at this first stage show that the possibility is rather remote.

Given that you are one of the lucky few to lose a reasonable amount of weight on a diet, you are now ready for the next and most difficult challenge. Once you have lost weight, you are faced with the problem of stopping the fat from returning. Here the picture for dieters is very bleak. The long-term success of diets is even worse than their very poor short-term success. The vast majority of people who lose weight regain all of that weight, usually within a year.

When faced with these unsavory but undeniable facts, disheartened aspirants to slenderness often make reference to someone they saw in a television commercial or magazine advertisement. Commercial diet propaganda has a fairly standard format. First there is the obligatory picture of a sad and lonely 250-pound Miss (it is always a Miss) Brown, slouching dejectedly in a shabby $2.50 dress purchased from a local thrift shop. Then there is the picture after Miss Brown became a purchaser of product X or a customer of studio Y. The second picture, which, in contrast to the first picture, is always in focus, shows a beaming, bolt-upright, maybe even Mrs. Smith (nee Brown) weighing in at 135 pounds and looking ravishing in a $2,500 designer original. "Why," asks the dieter, "can't this happen to me?"

What the slenderness vendors invariably fail to tell you is what Mrs. Smith looks like a year or so after being sprung from the diet program and her unmarried state. The bitter truth is that in a year or so, Mrs. Smith is very likely to have regained all the fat she lost. The long-term success rate of diets is even lower than the very low short-term success rate. Fewer than 5 percent of dieters manage to get slim and stay that way. Why do the other 95 percent of dieters, even those who are highly motivated and well informed, fail at dieting?

The common, facile, and rather useless explanation for failures at dieting is lack of willpower. The reason that this sort of explanation is useless is that it terminates the discourse by casting moral opprobrium. Further, it is not really an explanation at all. It is more of a restatement of the problem in moralistic terms. Moral judgments like this leave no place to go. However, if you must persist in this sort of analysis, there is a much more useful question to ask: Why is the fat person's will weak and how can you strengthen it? The ultimate poverty of notions such as willpower is well indicated by the fact that no one has ever bothered to suggest, short of reincarnation, how willpower might be improved.

The weak will of failed dieters is sometimes said to be due to the fact that they lack the proper motivation. However, motivational judgments are often little better than moral judgments. Most motivational analyses are just imprecise restatements of the initial problem. Where does the motivation come from? If fat people are not sufficiently motivated, how do we increase their motivation? Do we frighten them still more? I doubt that this is possible, since antifat feelings are already at near-panic levels.

If frightening fat people will not work, perhaps a more vigorous appeal to their sense of aesthetics would? Once again, I doubt that it is possible to make fatness much more ugly in the eyes of the general population. Many fat people already loathe their own bodies, and the revulsion of nonfat people for their fatter peers is all too often very thinly disguised.

The only two motives for dieting—health and beauty—have been so thoroughly wrung out that they offer virtually no prospects for improving dieters' motivation. In fact, the only evidence for lack of willpower or insufficient motivation of dieters is the failure of the diet. Pseudo explanations centered around vague notions such as willpower and motivation are circular and unproductive. They offer no real clues to understanding the problem. They are typically substitutes for understanding.

The present analysis has heretical implications. The conspicuous failure of diets is clearly not due to deficiencies in dead-end concepts such as willpower and motivation. Instead, the failure indicates the operation of very powerful basic biological forces. Overcoming these forces is the exception, and failure to overcome them is the norm. One could say that those few who do diet successfully are to be congratulated and esteemed much like an athlete who can run a four-minute mile. Alternately, successful dieters, like exceptional athletes, can be looked upon in a less evaluative manner as simply being exceptional.

The much more important issue is how one looks upon the

vast majority of dieters who fail in their attempts to lose weight. They should be considered in the same light as those of us who cannot run a four-minute mile or swim the English Channel. Failed dieters, like ordinary athletes, are statistically and physiologically normal. They are not physiologically, morally, or motivationally pathological. Failed dieters are the norm, whereas they are currently treated by others and by themselves as freaks and pariahs.

Viewed in this light, dieting takes on a new and vastly less sinister aspect. Like exceptional athletic pursuits, dieting should be looked upon as a challenge. If it interests you, then by all means try a diet or two. Who knows, you may be one of the rare genuine success stories. When diets are looked upon as a physiological experiment rather than as a test of one's moral fiber, many otherwise reluctant, would-be dieters may emerge. More important, the millions of failed dieters may at last have a chance at regaining the esteem robbed from them by an irrationally fatophobic society.

The potential benefits of this destigmatization of fat are enormous. First, it should dramatically reduce the large and unjustified load of stress with which we have burdened fat people. The benefits of this to their physical and mental health are inestimable. This should also have the effect of encouraging failed dieters to experiment with further diets on a "no-fault" basis. There is always the outside possibility that some new diet may just work where all others have failed.

There is a perilous balance to be maintained here. On one side there are considerations of truth. Weight-reducing diets have a very low success rate. To pretend otherwise to an aspiring dieter is both dishonest and ultimately counterproductive. On the other hand, there is the fact that there is a segment of the population who could genuinely benefit from weight reduction. These people should not be discouraged from pursuing weight loss. The position being developed in this book is an attempt to walk on both sides of the fence.

Second, removing the moral stigma from fat people should dramatically increase their involvement in many other aspects of healthy living. Defeated and depressed fat people who have not totally given up have, till now, concentrated with religious fervor on the energy content of their diets. As a direct result of their preoccupation with energy content, they have sadly neglected macronutrient composition.

In terms of importance to one's overall health status, macronutrient composition of a diet is at least as important as energy content. When diets fail, as they almost always do, fat people often abandon all hope of ever being healthy and adopt all the trappings of a maximally unhealthy life-style.

Failed dieters are prime candidates for taking up smoking, avoiding all forms of exercise and eating all of the wrong foods. They wallow in saturated fats and sugars. They avoid exercise, complex carbohydrates, and dietary fiber. There are real health gains to be reaped from exercising, reducing saturated fat intake, and increasing complex carbohydrate intake (see chapter 8). These may even have, as a secondary benefit, some weight-reducing properties. Up to now we have driven fat people away from healthy living. The present reevaluation should redress the balance and bring many fat people back into the fold of humanity.

No-Energy Diets

If a little energy restriction is good and a lot of energy restriction is better, then total starvation should be best. Starvation is, of course, the ultimate diet. With no energy intake, patients must live entirely on their own energy stores. As a result, total starvation produces the largest and fastest weight loss. Since fat contains 5,000 kcal per lb and the average person needs about 2,600 kcal per day, total starvation should produce a loss of about 5 lb per week.

It does not require a mathematician to calculate that losing weight at a rate of 5 lb/week can consume over 250 lb/year. The maximal reduction in energy expenditure that might occur in response to starvation could reduce the starvation weight loss to as little as 125 lb/year. In other words, even in the face of maximal energetic compensation, starvation will produce massive weight loss.

All this sounds pretty good, which is why various commercial organizations like to use starvation on their customers. Starvation produces dramatic weight loss, and this sells more fat people on buying their product or subscribing to their service. Alas, as is so often the case, the commercial interests may be good for business, but they are not so good for the customer.

Another way starvation is sold, is on the basis that it is ultimately not only faster but easier than normal dieting. The reason why starvation produces faster weight loss is obvious, but the reason why it is alleged to be easier than normal dieting requires some explanation. Starvation, because it mobilizes fat reserves, releases large amounts of ketones into the circulation. This process is called *ketosis*. All sorts of wonderful properties have been ascribed to ketones and ketosis.

Actually, ketosis is not the simple result of mobilizing fat reserves. It is also dependent on a lack of concurrent breakdown of carbohydrates. Starvation advocates claim that ketosis reduces the sensation of hunger. They are usually quick to point out that starvation-induced satiety does not occur until you have been starving for a few days. According to its proponents, starvation offers the promise of rapid weight loss with only transient and minimal discomfort due to hunger.

All this sounds too good to be true. It is not only untrue, it is utter nonsense. One of the most striking characteristics of starving people is that they feel very hungry. They are ravaged by hunger night and day. If hunger were not so dreadfully unpleasant, the starving legions of the world would be thanking us for giving them the opportunity to starve.

Starving people may be able to pretend that they are not hungry and, in the short term, they may even be able to be persuaded that this is true. However, starvation does produce real hunger, and real hunger does not just go away. Anyone who tells you something different is either terribly ignorant or wants to sell you something (this combination is often a package deal). There is a terminal stage of starvation where the victim becomes quite oblivious to everything including hunger, but this occurs just before death. One of the causes of the delirium that occurs in starvation is the toxic effect that ketone bodies have on the brain. The toxic effects of ketones are largely responsible for the coma that results from untreated diabetes.

Yet another mythical attraction of starvation is that it produces a unique "high" that enhances spirituality. This is part of the reason why fasting is a common part of many religions. One of the most remarkable features of the human species is that we often respond the way we are told to respond, no matter how inappropriate that response is. Many substances that produce only minor effects are reported to produce various highs when the users expect it. We are suckers for placebos.

The placebo effect is a common thread throughout medicine. Fasting usually produces a feeling of giddiness and weakness. The giddiness results from the inability to properly adjust blood pressure to changes in posture. It is also partly due to the toxic effects ketone bodies have on the brain. In the very naive, or in true believers, these uncomfortable sensations might be reported as a high. If a normal person stands up suddenly, he or she may experience a brief period of dizziness as blood drains out of the brain. This phenomenon of "postural hypotension" is exaggerated by starvation.

In the light of day and stripped of the influence of suggestion, the high produced by fasting appears to be about as pleasant as that produced by a rapid change in posture or by a common virus. If weakness and disorientation are your trip, fasting may be for you. Very few fasters remain enthusiastic about fasting after trying it more than a few times. One negative effect of starvation is that the fasting causes the loss of both fat and protein. Unfortunately, the weight gains that follow starvation are almost exclusively fat. Repeated starvation cycles can seriously reduce your muscle mass and increase fat mass. This, in itself, could make further attempts at weight loss even more difficult.

A recent source of enthusiasm for fasting comes from reports that intermittent starvation increases the life span of laboratory mice and rats. Thus slenderizing became not just the path to beauty and health but also the path to eternal youth. The laboratory results were supported by reports of extremely long life expectancies in a number of remote areas of the world where food is in chronic short supply. In rugged, mountainous areas, such as the Andes and the Caucasus, life expectancies have been said to be as much as twice what the rest of the world considers normal.

Propelled by this apparent alliance of laboratory results and human life expectancy data, thousands have submitted themselves to various starvation regimens. The search for eternal youth has been given a new lease on life. Unfortunately, neither pillar of this new fad will support much weight. First, whereas starvation may increase the life expectancy of caged rodents fed a uniform, monotonous diet, it is not at all clear whether it would have any beneficial effect on animals in more natural settings. There are no data suggesting that starvation increases the life span of free-running rodents that select a varied diet. So, it is not even clear whether the beneficial effects of intermittent starvation apply to rats and mice in general. It is a greater leap to say that these findings apply to other rodents.

It is an immense leap to apply these results to humans. Compared with humans, rodents have extremely high metabolic rates. They have been described as living in a metabolic "fast lane." However, this criticism is essentially theoretical. The real question becomes, Is there any evidence that food restriction increases human longevity? Until these laboratory data from animals are shown to apply to humans, statements that starvation increases longevity can only be considered to be groundless speculation.

There have been reports that suggest that semistarvation increases human life expectancy in the Andes, the Caucasus, and so on. Unfortunately, these titillating reports turn out to be uniformly ill founded. They appear to be a joint product of observer gullibility and the confused state of records that typically exists away from mainstream civilization. Chronic malnutrition does lead to reduced intellectual abilities.

Thus far we have determined that hunger is rather unpleasant and that it is not likely to increase longevity. However, starvation has other effects that go far beyond mere discomfort. A starving person may burn up protein instead of fat, and this use of essential protein may have some very dangerous consequences. It now appears that, in many cases, starvation produces permanent muscle damage. This starvation-induced muscle damage (myopathy) may not be reversed by refeeding. One of the more vulnerable organs for starvation-induced myopathy is the heart. Starvation may literally make you eat your heart out.

In addition to the direct assault on the heart muscle described above, starvation provides an equally serious indirect threat to cardiovascular health. The whole idea of a fast is to use up fat reserves. The only way that fat can be shed is by using it as fuel. Consequently, a fast is a 100 percent saturated-fat (that is, animal fat) diet. One of the consistent findings of modern nutrition is that a diet high in saturated fats is very unhealthy. Just why this is the case is not certain, but the fact remains that it is. The risk associated with a diet high in saturated fats is particularly serious for anyone with heart problems.

The fact that starvation is really just a 100 percent fat (your own fat) diet also illuminates some of the other absurd claims made by starvation advocates. There is a common belief that fasting has a purgative or cleansing effect on the blood. This is yet another one of the absurd claims in this area that is still given wide credence. It can be debunked quite simply.

As pointed out above, starvation is really just a total-saturated-fat diet. You wouldn't expect a total-fat diet to be particularly cleansing, and it's not. If anything, starvation places an increased load on the liver and kidneys. Pretty much the only things purged by a fast are valuable vitamins, minerals, and proteins. More radical claims that fasting is a cure for serious diseases such as epilepsy and cancer are just cruel nonsense.

In addition to the dangers described above, there are many other serious potential complications of total starvation. Consequently, if you even contemplate starvation, it should be remembered that it must only be done in a hospital ward under proper medical supervision. Quasi-medical weight-loss clinics rarely have adequate expertise to cope with the unexpected and unpredictable contingencies that can arise during such a drastic treatment. This, of course, makes starvation very expensive and practical only for that small minority with an abundance of time to spare.

There have been reported deaths due to starvation. Starvation-induced death is sudden and without any warning. It may even occur in healthy, young people. Its precise cause is not clear, but its occurrence is indisputable. The fact that many people still persist with this mad treatment shows how desperate fat people have become.

As if this list of dangers were not enough, there is still another major criticism of starvation as a treatment for fatness. This criticism is not one of potential dangers, but one of efficacy. After the fast is over, the victims of starvation rapidly regain all their lost weight and then some. There are several studies showing that, as a treatment for fatness, starvation is worse than no treatment at all.

Fasting appears to increase the likelihood of getting still fatter. It appears that starvation, whether it is acute or intermittently repeated, shapes up your metabolism to better fight subsequent attempts at losing weight. Starvation may even reset your body-weight set-point at a higher level. This is the basis for the seemingly paradoxical statement that dieting makes you fat. Not only is starvation extremely dangerous, it is also thoroughly counterproductive.

Low-Carbohydrate Diets

If there is a single substance cast in the role of the main culprit in fatness it has to be carbohydrates. *Pasta, pizza, bread, potatoes,* and (gasp!) *sugar* are such guilt-laden terms that their very mention causes weight watchers to blanch. Since the vast majority of human diets have carbohydrates as their main ingredient, any low-carbohydrate diet necessarily becomes a high-fat and/or high-protein diet.

Fats also come in for a lot of criticism, but not nearly as much as carbohydrates. Almost all diets place bans on carbohydrates, while few make fats taboo. In fact, as we will see below, one of the most popular diets of all time is a high-fat diet. Further, there is an abundance of high-protein diets.

Nobody takes up cudgels against proteins; few take up cudgels against fat; yet most in the diet world condemn carbohydrates. Carbohydrates are seen as being a particularly indulgent and nutritionally worthless foodstuff. Proteins are absolutely necessary, and fats are tolerated, but carbohydrates are a frivolous excess.

The anticarbohydrate lobby sees carbohydrates as being worse than a simple indulgence. Some diet messiahs have gone even further than blaming excess weight on carbohydrates. They maintain that demon hunger itself is due to eating carbohydrates. There have been a number of popular diets that maintain that you can eat limitless fat and protein, but as long as you abstain from carbohydrates, you will lose weight and not feel hungry. The meat and blubber diet of Eskimos is said to be their secret to slenderness.

This is a complete and groundless fabrication. Any diet that promises weight loss without reducing energy intake is a hustle. Water does not flow uphill, and weight is not lost if energy intake is greater than energy expenditure. If you eat much fat, your energy intake cannot possibly be less than your energy expenditure. Eskimos tend to be fat. Slender Eskimos are either sick or starving. Like most sensible people, Eskimos do not choose to be thin.

One of the most commercially successful of the low-carbohydrate diets was the Drinking Man's Diet. This diet was first widely aired in a tiny pamphlet that was largely made up of tables taken from U.S. government publications. The text was conspicuous by its relative absence. The lack of text was no real drawback, since the authors did not really have much to say. A lack of intellectual stimulation has never hurt the sales performance of any diet.

The Drinking Man's Diet was a runaway best-seller because of its unusual "eat, drink, and be merry" approach. Eating, drinking, and being merry, of course, specifically excluded carbohydrates. Much of its appeal was the fact that, in contrast to virtually every other diet, it was not a renouncement of pleasure.

The Drinking Man's Diet clearly bucked the mainstream diet themes of purge, penance, and privation. With all this going for it, there is only one real criticism of this diet. It does not work. On the other hand, there is a not entirely facetious argument that if you are going to fail, you might as well have a good time doing it.

Carbohydrates are first and foremost fun. The leader of this frivolous band is unquestionably sugar. Sugar is the only taste that humans universally like from birth. All other tastes require a substantial amount of learning. It should come as no surprise that most diet merchants give sugar a high priority on their hit list.

The first high-fat diet was a direct reaction to the perceived evils of sugar and its fellow carbohydrates. In the mid nineteenth century, the great French physiologist Claude Bernard discovered it was possible to control diabetes by restricting sugar intake. The English ear surgeon, William Harvey, applied this logic to his fat patient, William Banting (who had an earache). Harvey put Banting on a diet based on mutton, bacon, and other meats. This diet specifically minimized all forms of carbohydrates.

It is not really clear whether Banting lost the earache that was the original target of the diet. However, Banting did lose weight. Earache or no, Banting published his "miracle cure." Banting's "Letter on Corpulence" was the first successful diet publication, and he became the first diet guru.

Dr. Harvey disappeared from the scene, but the British term for dieting, *Banting,* remains to this day. Significantly, Banting's trade was coffin making. This established the precedent that to be a diet guru it is preferable that you know nothing about dieting, medicine, or physiology. Along with the term *Banting,* this precedent is the main legacy of the first popular diet.

The high-fat, low-carbohydrate diet first exploited by Banting was reincarnated as the DuPont diet in the 1950s. The DuPont diet had about the same flimsy rationale as the nineteenth-century original, but it did add one new and essential ingredient—the catch phrase. In order to fleece the flock, you have to get them into the tent. Given the short attention span and aversion to thinking evidenced by the general public, necessity mothered the catch phrase. The DuPont diet advocated, "Eat fat and think thin."

The most elementary considerations of energy balance indicate that if you really eat fat, you may be able to think thin, but that is about as close to getting thin as you are likely to get. Like all of those diets before and afterward, the DuPont diet was not particularly concerned with whether or not it produced weight loss. It's prime consideration, like that of virtually all diets, was the jingle of the cash register. To keep the cash flow up requires that you capitalize on your apparent successes and dismiss or, better yet, totally ignore the failures. If someone fails using your product, it's his or her fault, not yours. This lucrative, if ethically dubious, practice remains the industry standard. Some standard, some industry.

This same wheel was yet again rediscovered by Dr. Herman Taller, who cashed in with his best-seller *Calories Don't Count* in the early 1960s. Taller espoused his "new nutrition principles," which essentially said that to lose fat, you must eat fat. The title of the book was no less absurd than its underlying logic. To say that calories don't count is akin to saying that gravity is irrelevant.

Taller's twist on this already old theme was to stress the importance of unsaturated fats. Unsaturated fat have less potential than the saturated fats in meat and dairy products for raising cholesterol levels. This was rather more sensible than what the public was told by the earlier high-fat diets. By this time the medical community was already placing cholesterol in the pillory. Taller claimed that unsaturated fats stimulate the release of a fat-destroying hormone. Taller's brand of hucksterism was a runaway success until he attracted the interest of U.S. federal authorities. They were less than enthusiastic about his gospel. He was convicted of fraud and drug offenses.

By this time it should come as no great surprise that these thoroughly discredited ideas were dredged up still another time. In this case the beneficiary of the public's gullibility and attendant generosity was Dr. Robert Atkins. He threw in the wrinkle of measuring ketosis (which is an index of fat utilization in the absence of carbohydrates). His diet was, in another sense, a throwback, since it advocated eating large quantities of saturated fats.

The medical community was aghast, since it had been working steadily to convince the public of the dangers of saturated fats and their downstream product, cholesterol. Atkins, too, came to some grief at the hands of a skeptical judiciary. However, his wings were only trimmed, not clipped. We will see below that he and his bank balance have soared again, this time on the wings of fructose.

It may well be that the whole issue of dietary regulation of serum cholesterol levels has been seriously distorted. There is little doubt that high serum cholesterol levels are a very bad sign in anyone with cardiovascular problems. Where the controversy occurs is with respect to the origins and treatment of high serum cholesterol levels. It appears that most of the body's cholesterol is synthesized in the liver, and it may be largely independent of dietary cholesterol intake. On the other hand, this is still an equivocal issue, and there is certainly no suggestion that reducing cholesterol intake has any negative effects. Further, there is growing evidence that although cholesterol intake may not directly affect serum cholesterol levels, high intake of saturated fats may well impair the body's mechanisms for dealing with cholesterol. This would mean that the warnings about dietary cholesterol were essentially right, but for the wrong reasons.

The most recent manifestation of the anticarbohydrate hysteria is the fructose craze. Fructose has been elevated to the status of a saint among the unholy group of sugars. The illogic surrounding fructose is formidable. The fructose nonsense is slightly more insidious than some of the other hustles, since it is shrouded in pseudo-endocrine terms.

The advocates of salvation through fructose claim that fructose, unlike glucose, enters directly into muscle cells and does not stimulate the hunger-producing hormone insulin. Both of these pivotal statements are wrong. Fructose, like all other sugars, does not enter muscle cells until it is converted into glucose. In fact, fructose does not do much of anything until it is converted into glucose. After fructose is converted into glucose, it has all of glucose's normal effects, including mobilizing insulin. To put it simply, fructose is really the wolf glucose in cheap clothing.

Actually fructose is not clad in particularly cheap clothing. The fact that the claims made for it range from hyperbole to outright fantasy makes it expensive at any price. Dr. Atkins cashed in on this one, too, with his superenergy diets. Considering the fact that fructose is really just preglucose, the only particular spring it is likely to put in anyone's step is in that of Atkins and cohorts on the way to the bank. Since it encourages high fat, it is just as bad as all the others in this category.

The numerous low- or no-carbohydrate diets should be seen for what they really are. They are inevitably either high-fat and/or high-protein diets. Although the vast majority of contemporary nutritionists recommend that most people reduce their protein intake, it is by no means clear whether high protein intake, as such, has harmful effects. At the very least, substantially reducing protein intake appears to have no harmful effects at all. So if a low-carbohydrate diet were really just a high-protein diet, it might be relatively harmless. However, this is almost never the case. The elimination of carbohydrates from the diet almost inevitably involves an increase in fat intake.

The situation with respect to the effects of fat intake on health is becoming increasingly clear. Most nutritionists agree that typical Western diets have far too much fat in them. Typical diets in most developed countries have about 40 to 60 percent of their total energy value as fat. This is probably two to three times more than the optimal value, which may be as low as 20 percent.

High dietary intake of fats, particularly saturated fats, is clearly associated with high levels of blood cholesterol. High blood levels of cholesterol and related lipids are unequivocally associated with serious heart and vascular problems. In fact, it appears that much of the health hazard attributed to fatness is likely due to the high cholesterol levels seen in fat people and not to the fatness itself.

Although the composition of a diet in terms of macronutrients (that is, carbohydrate, fat, or protein) is irrelevant to weight loss, it is important to overall health status. Particularly in fat people, any increase in cholesterol is to be avoided. The best available data suggest that high serum cholesterol levels produce a 250 percent increase in the likelihood of fat people dying from cardiovascular disease. Any high-fat diet has the potential to significantly exacerbate the health problems of fat people. Moreover, high-fat diets are highly unlikely to bring about substantial or permanent weight loss. Consequently, increasing dietary fat must be looked upon as foolish or even dangerous. Thus low-carbohydrate diets can only be seen as bad medicine.

The low-carbohydrate diets illustrate another important principle of the diet business. Popular diet books are invariably largely composed of highly structured menus. This illustrates the point that the desperate dieting public wants to be told what to do. Tell them firmly enough and often enough and as long as you promise weight loss, they'll follow you over cliffs. At the same time, the menus and tables out of which most diet books are fabricated suggest that the author doesn't really have much to say. The conceptual framework underlying most diets is pathetic. The fact that the public continues to gobble this swill up shows how desperate the situation is.

To be a successful diet merchant you have to be a demagogue. The sales pitch is ultimately the only thing that differentiates one diet from another, since none of them works. Alternately, one could maintain the position that any low-energy diet will work if you only adhere to it. In the final analysis, of course, the problem is one of failure to follow diets. This is not just a minor hitch. It is the reason that no diet really works and why most diets could work.

If you keep up the patter long enough, your acolytes never have to think at all. It doesn't matter much what you tell them as long as it keeps them coming back for more. If you can't give them real medicine, at least keep them hypnotized with babble. Rediscover the square wheel and give it a catchy new name and you are on your way.

Most dieters appear to be kept going by the bliss of abject surrender to a tantalizing promise. It certainly isn't weight loss that keeps them going. There just isn't enough of that to go around. When all the frills and flapdoodle are stripped from any diet, the same specter is revealed. Something that just doesn't work. It is either nonsense from the start or it is basically all right, if only it could be adhered to. The bottom line is, alas, the same: The dieter is out of luck.

Liquid-Protein Diets

The illogical extreme of minimizing carbohydrates is to eliminate them altogether. If you eliminate carbohydrates, the diet has to be entirely composed of fats and/or protein. Since high-fat diets have a number of problems of their own, the obvious way out is an all-protein diet.

Many high-protein diets have been based on lean meat, but even lean meat has some of the dreaded high-energy fat in it. Why not eliminate fat and carbohydrate altogether? This, of course, leaves only protein. The only way to have an all-protein diet is to liquefy proteins and purge everything else along the way. Liquid-protein diets also avoid the dieters' perennial problem of having to choose among various foods. The easiest way to deal with choice is to eliminate it entirely. Liquid-protein diets were presented as convenient, entirely self-contained solutions to weight loss.

Liquid-protein diets also claim to address the problem of protein destruction that occurs when energy intake is restricted. Remember that the ideal situation during negative energy balance is that the dieter only uses fat for energy. However, this ideal is almost never achieved. Dieters often sacrifice a lot of their own protein on stringent diets. The loss of muscle can be a minor problem, or, in extreme cases, the sacrifice of heart muscle can be life threatening. The liquid-protein diets offers the possibility of providing so much protein that the dieter would have no need to sacrifice his or her own protein. Not only that, but protein has acquired a saintly status in folk nutrition. It's the reason why top athletes always have a steak before a strenuous event, why lumberjacks are red-meat eaters, and so on.

The arguments in favor of liquid protein diets followed above are virtually entirely incorrect. This diet is one of the most dangerous diets ever to achieve widespread acceptance. It is important to add that in spite of all its nutritional inadequacies the liquid protein diet is no more effective in bringing about weight loss than any other radically unbalanced diet.

A common feature of all unbalanced diets is that they cause a net reduction in energy intake. This reduction does not reflect any diet magic. It is merely due to the boredom and occasional nausea attendant on eating any unbalanced diet. No matter how much you like any food, that food by itself becomes boring and unpalatable. The more nutritionally inadequate the food, the sooner the boredom effect sets in. This sort of short-term trickery produces, at best, short-term results. You cannot live for long on an unbalanced diet. Short-term illusory weight loss is no foundation on which to build permanent weight loss.

Liquid-protein preparations are not complete diets. This should come as no great surprise, since the biggest seller in this field was made from animal connective tissue and hide. This stuff was just one step away from glue. The bizarre dietary imbalance created by eating only protein is compounded by the flushing out of vitamins and minerals. This diet also tends to increase serum cholesterol, which is particularly dangerous for patients with any sort of cardiovascular problems. The lack of carbohydrates also tends to cause ketosis. Ketosis is particularly dangerous during pregnancy. There are data showing that it may cause mental retardation in the newborn.

These criticisms have been dismissed by saying that the drawbacks of the all-protein diets are only peripheral niggles. If you want to make an omelet, you must break eggs. This type of sophistry, however, ignores a couple of important points. First, these wonder diets do not work. A calorie is a calorie no matter who its parents are. There is no evidence that the high-protein diets are any better in terms of facilitating weight loss than any of the competition. We already know that the competition is pretty worthless.

Most nutritionists are coming around to the belief that carbohydrate intake should be increased, not decreased. There is nothing at all magical about protein. Athletes who eat a steak before the big event are way out of date. Sports nutritionists are nearly unanimous in the view that a high-carbohydrate meal is much more effective in building up muscle reserves of glycogen. It is these reserves that the athletes must draw upon during exertion.

Further, high-carbohydrate diets with their attendant high content of dietary fiber are likely to be far kinder to your digestive tract. Diets low in fiber (that is, high-protein diets) are associated with cancers of the lower digestive tract. There is even some, albeit equivocal, indication that high-fiber diets may produce a greater degree of satiety for a given level of energy intake. This is essentially the opposite of the position developed by the protein lobby. They claim that high-protein diets also have a high satiety value. They fail, however, to back up their claim with anything other than rhetoric.

To call the liquid-protein diets worthless is not really correct or fair. They are less than worthless. Liquid-protein diets cause occasional irregularities in the heart rhythm even in healthy young people. As a result of their tendency to cause electrocardiological anomalies, liquid-protein diets have been implicated in scores of deaths in the United States alone. The international death toll of this madness has yet to be determined.

Fortunately, the adverse publicity and litigation surrounding this type of diet seems to have struck home. Lethality is pretty frightening, even for the fat desperadoes. Super-protein diets, liquid or otherwise, are now pretty much a spent force in the marketplace. However, given the almost inevitably cyclic pattern of diet madness, it is likely that they will reappear before long. Of course, born-again liquid-protein diets will appear in slightly different clothing. At that time they will be hailed (by their promoters) as a "new and unbelievable" breakthrough. The promoters will be half right.

Lunatic-Fringe Diets

The above discussion by no means exhausts the list of diets currently in use. It merely represents some of the major trends. Perhaps it does a disservice to the legitimate diet industry by concentrating on the quackier end of the spectrum. There are good, sensible diets around. You don't need a guru to lead you to them. To lose weight, you must achieve a prolonged state of negative energy balance. This is the aim of any good diet. Unfortunately, good diets are ultimately little better for producing weight loss than are the quack diets. Their conceptual soundness does not make them work. The likelihood of a sound diet working is only marginally better than that of a quack diet. One conspicuous advantage of a good diet is that it harms little other than your self-esteem. Similarly, good diets are likely to be advocated by medical professionals, who really do have your best interests at heart. Quack diets are typically sold by quacks, who have little or no medical knowledge and even less interest in your well-being. Most quacks are only in it for the money. Even the well-intentioned quacks are dangerous. When you seek help, see a doctor, not a guru.

There is a substantial segment of the population who seek weight loss through diets that belong to what I would call the lunatic fringe. It is debatable at what point quackery degenerates into lunatic fringery. I suppose the critical issue is whether the diet makes any physiological sense at all. Most of the quack diets above have a central element that is based on some demonstrated physiological principle. This core truth is usually distorted beyond all reason in pursuit of the holy grail (weight loss) and/or greed.

The lunacy that abounds on the periphery of the diet business appears to be motivated by both greed and stupidity. In fact, my relegating these diets to the periphery of the diet business may be wishful thinking. All too many of them appear to be getting center-stage billing. At least a hundred diets have claimed to be "the last diet you will ever need." The world clearly has needed none of these.

The claims for the lunatic-fringe diets extend far beyond simple weight loss. Destroy cellulite, rejuvenate, improve your sex life are but a few of the outrageous claims made by diet hucksters. Of course, all these miracles are preferably performed without any inconvenience to the dieter. If you are going to have a miracle, you might as well have one that is easy. Being easy never hurts the marketability of any diet. It may not do much for credibility, but that usually takes a backseat, since most dieters will believe almost anything.

Like the more mainstream, slightly quacky diets, the lunatic-fringe diets are totally dependent on avoiding any rigorous test of their claims. If there is any evidence used to support their claims, it is invariably either anecdotal or totally fabricated. Frequently, the claims are supported by no evidence at all. To swallow this drivel requires a religious faith in the guru and a total suppression of common sense. The claims of the quack brigade cannot stand and will not tolerate any independent evaluation.

However, in the final analysis the soundness of the concepts of any diet are irrelevant. So, too, are the flimsy results or lack of any results that they use to support their claims. It is not impossible that some crazy idea could just be the final solution that everyone is looking for. Irrespective of its origin, there is one characteristic of the genuine wonder diet that no one could miss: positive results!

Should this genuine wonder diet appear, it would offer clear and irrefutable results. It would work. The knowledge of these results would spread like wildfire, and the rest of the diet industry would wither away overnight. The hard sell and hyperbole that are the hallmarks of the diet marketplace would be entirely unnecessary. Anyone who really has something worthwhile to sell you does not have to twist your arm.

The lunatic-fringe diets offer mindless concepts and have no real secrets to weight loss. Another distressing aspect of the lunatic fringe is the fact that it tends to drag the whole issue off into fantasy land, where no solutions are ever likely to be found. Ignorance and superstition breed further ignorance and superstition. That is about all that these diets have to offer.

In the late twentieth century, public education has reached into more corners of the world than most people had imagined possible. At the same time, absurd and superstitious beliefs are given more public credence than ever before. In some areas this craziness is fairly harmless and should be tolerated, but in nutrition and public health it hurts a lot of people.

If the lunatic fringe needed a mascot, it would have to be the grapefruit. The humble grapefruit has played a central role in an astonishing array of crazy diets. As a result, international grapefruit sales skyrocketed. In the United States there was an acute grapefruit shortage in the late 1970s. The hype has it that grapefruits contain some wonder substance that "melts away fat." It's amazing how tenacious this fiction is. In some circles eating a grapefruit, particularly outside of breakfast hours, is still looked upon with sacramental awe.

As is always the case, if a little is good, then lots must be a lot better. People were (and still are) encouraged to gorge themselves on grapefruits as an active assault on fat. Alas, it is all hokum. Eating huge quantities of grapefruit produces little more than diarrhea. Diarrhea will produce some transient fluid loss, but it leaves your fat untouched. As much as you might like the idea, fat is not lost through excretion. Fat can only be lost when it is used as energy, and that can only occur during negative energy balance. There is no way to circumvent this immutable truth. The grapefruit is no magic road to negative energy balance, or even to diarrhea.

There is nothing at all special about the grapefruit. It is a rather tasty, fairly low-energy fruit that is quite high in vitamin C. As for its containing a miracle "fat blaster" or "blob buster," it is no different in this respect than an apple, bread, or butter. The hustlers can puff and they can bellow, but a calorie is still a calorie no matter what sort of package it comes in. Being a slightly bitter fruit perhaps made the grapefruit a better placebo. It's strange that no one (yet) has bestowed such miraculous properties upon pizza. Just imagine, "purge pounds through pizza," "amazing secrets of those slender Neapolitan housewives," "anchovies eat cellulite."

Now that cellulite has reared its ugly head, it is time that we gave it some consideration. Cellulite is that rather puckered stuff sometimes found on fat deposits. Since cellulite is rare in young people, it is feared as a sign of old age. Perhaps this is why cellulite is generally held to be even uglier than ordinary fat. The fear and loathing of cellulite is compounded by the fact that it appears to be even more resistant to destruction than regular fat. Cellulite is essentially just ordinary fat, and the detested puckering is due to the presence of unusually large amounts of connective tissue. The reason for the proliferation of connective tissue in ordinary fat deposits is not known. There is, as yet, no apparent function for cellulite.

Magical diets have been invented to cure almost every human woe, from fallen arches to stuttering. Consequently, it should come as no surprise that there are diets specifically addressed to attacking cellulite. One anticellulite crusader attacked cellulite by first inventing a whole new and mythical structure for it. He said that it was a gel-like combination of fat, water, and wastes. The key was in the recurring theme of "toxic wastes," a perennial favorite among food fetishists. Cellulite, like any other fat, is not a storehouse of wastes, toxic or otherwise.

Given a mythical structure and mythical origins, it is easy to design a diet to attack the myth. In this case the assault on cellulite was led by troops of fresh vegetables and fruits. Somehow these foods were assumed to be effective in ridding the body of the fictitious "toxic wastes." This sort of diet may destroy the mythical cellulite, but it certainly has no effect at all on real cellulite.

The gullibility of the public was sorely tried in another anti-cellulite book. This "amazing" publication tells you how to find cellulite, how it comes about, and just how horrid and ugly it is. Then they have the effrontery to tell you that they do not advocate any specific diet to get rid of it! They assume that you already know enough to eat sensibly, so keep it up! At least you have to congratulate them on truth in packaging. The most amazing thing about the diet is that many thousands of people paid to be told that they were not going to be helped by the book. P. T. Barnum seriously underestimated the birth rate of suckers.

The unsavory truth about cellulite is that its structure is fairly well known, but its function remains an enigma. More important, there appears to be no way to get rid of it. No dietary or any other means has been shown to have any effect at all on cellulite. You can diet it, knead it, pummel it, anoint it, and assault it in a dozen other ways. The end result is the same. If you have cellulite today, you are certain to have it tomorrow.

There is another cluster of crazy diets that claim you can nibble your way to slenderness. These diets are based upon the following pseudo logic. First is the remarkable observation that barnyard animals are not fat. They say that the secret of the slenderness of the beasts of the barnyard is the fact that they eat almost continually. As a result, their energy intake is very close to their energy expenditure. According to the nibbling advocates, if humans were to follow the example of our barnyard brethren, our fat would melt away. All these diets advocate splitting food intake into a large number of snacks or nibbles, as opposed to the small number of discrete meals we normally eat.

These diets are laughably wrong in almost every respect. First, barnyard animals are not necessarily thin. When the competition for food is not too fierce, barnyard beasts are quite adept at getting fat. The reason they eat continually is that normally they have to in order to get enough food to survive. They are not slim because they eat continually, rather they eat continually because they are slim. If you give barnyard animals an abundant supply of high-energy-content food they develop clear-cut meal patterns and gain weight. So, the fundamental observation on which these diets are based is incorrect. Applying this misinformation to humans is doubly absurd.

The only way these diets have any hope of working is through reducing total energy intake. Indeed, underneath all the nibbling nonsense, most of these diets simply turn out to be fairly standard low-energy diets. There are no magical benefits to be reaped from eating a lot of meals because, as we already know, the only way out of fatness is through achieving a prolonged state of negative energy balance. There is no real mystery to this. Nibbling is simply another dietary red herring.

One of the core themes of the lunatic fringe is the ageless quest to get something for nothing. If there is one giant fact to emerge from examining the diet literature, it is that if real weight loss is possible at all, it will inevitably be a very arduous task. Consequently, one of the common diet sales pitches is that with method A or product B you can lose weight easily, quickly, and with no personal effort—"no willpower required." That would be real magic. Needless to say, there have been plenty of efforts to woo the dieter's wallet in this manner. When there is money in magic, magicians multiply faster than the rabbits in their hats. The diet business is full of those who can most charitably be called magicians.

One of these forms of dietary magic is based upon our body clock. It is a well-accepted truth of physiology that most physiological processes wax and wane regularly over each twenty-four-hour period. Chronobiology is the study of these biological rhythms. Merchants of various "body-clock" diets maintain that you can eat whatever you want as long as you eat it early in the day. They brandish the time-worn cliché of "scientific proof" to support their claims. As far as I know, nobody has ever seen such proof. It must be really hot stuff.

Once again, like all of the others, this type of diet is long on promises and short on results. It is a shortcut to nowhere. Energetically speaking, you can't get something for nothing, no matter how much you may deserve it. The basic laws of physiology will not be circumvented by vacant patter. That is all these chronobiological diets have to offer. They muddy the good name of a new and legitimate branch of physiology. They would never be endorsed by a serious chronobiologist.

There have been several diets that have been billed as nine-day wonders. It is not always clear whether the nine days is meant to indicate the duration of the diet or the expected duration of public belief in their twaddle. The catch phrase of one of these wonders was CBO (calorie burnout). It also cashed in on another lucrative promise. It made the observation that with normal diets your weight is lost in a rather indiscriminate manner. They promised that their diet would target specific "problem areas" and melt them away. Presumably this diet attacked the belly and double chin while sparing the breast and the more succulent parts of the bottom.

This laudable aim is pure fantasy. When you burn up fat during a period of negative energy balance, your body is completely oblivious as to where it gets the fat from. To expect otherwise is like saying that you can get your car to use the gas from one side of the tank and not the other. As if that drivel were not enough to ensure their financial immortality, they added still more hype. They claimed that over time their calorie burnout gathered momentum sufficient to allow dieters to resume gorging themselves and at the same time continue to lose weight. This miracle weight loss was presumably brought about through the agency of the tooth fairy and the mayor of Atlantis.

Corn is as good an ingredient as any to use as the basis of a hairbrain diet. It is interesting that so many diets have isolated a particular food element either as the road to slenderness and salvation or as the road to pounds and perdition. One of the more enterprising of these diet fabricators didn't settle for just one panacea, she opted for a miracle combination of four. This holy host consisted of lecithin, vinegar, kelp, and vitamin B_6.

The rationale behind the choice of these life-saving ingredients makes the Great Pyramid Corn Diet look pretty sound.

Lecithin is an emulsifier that is added to fatty foods to enhance the digestion of fats. Why it would facilitate weight loss remains a mystery of pyramidal proportions. The rationale for drinking vinegar is that oil and vinegar don't mix! Thus she not only displays an abysmal ignorance of physiology, but she has also obviously never made a salad dressing. The use of kelp and vitamin B_6 rests on foundations that are every bit as fanciful as their other two partners in this fatuous alliance. This diet constitutes a much greater assault on credibility than it does on fat.

This list of lunatic diets could go on forever. It is hard to pick up a fashion, health, or life-style magazine without some new diet silliness leaping out at you. The popular press continues to promulgate the false notion that weight loss is fairly simple once you have found the right formula. If weight loss were at all simple, there would be hardly any fat people. The media compound their guilt by their blind and wholesale acceptance of the equally false notion that weight loss is a generally desirable goal. Only a small fraction of those who attempt to lose weight could genuinely profit from weight loss. The horns of this dilemma continue to gore millions of people around the world.

CHAPTER 6

FIGHTING FAT WITH EXERCISE

The use of exercise as a means to lose weight is a very emotional issue. Broadly speaking, the community falls into two camps on the exercise issue. There is the "life be in it" group, who find music in the twang of stretched ligaments. They see exercise as a panacea and as a purgative for the physical and moral decay that is eating away at the core of the Western world. Exercise is for them a fundamental moral issue.

Exercise as a Moral Issue

Like other moral evangelists, the jockstrap elite feels no qualms about inflicting their value system on the rest of the world. They won't settle for having everyone else march in line, they want a brisk jog instead. Their brand of organized self-flagellation is the only road to producing the *uebermensch* (superman). Their heads are filled with visions of bronzed legions of Adonis youths, muscles rippling in the sun. They see clean air, the eradication of disease, and eternal youth, all within our grasp, hovering above an aerobic chalice.

The other camp holds almost diametrically opposed views. Their contempt for the lure of liniment and perspiration is obvious. They see their bodies as being tough-engineered by evolution to withstand the slings and arrows of modern life without having to scurry off to a gym every day. Real men don't wear jockstraps. Their clearly defensive posture is partly dictated by the fact that they harbor a lurking suspicion that the other camp may just be right. Both of these extreme views are incorrect. Each conceals what exercise can and cannot do for you. Like so many of the views in the fat and fitness marketplace, they are largely based upon untenable, if tenacious, assumptions. It is time these assumptions were examined more closely.

The initial logic of the exercise advocates seems very straightforward. The only way to lose weight is to expend more energy than you take in. This simple rule is to weight loss what the law of gravity is to high jumping. There is no way to get around it, no matter how much you might want to. The problems associated with trying to reduce the input end of the energy-balance equation (dieting) were discussed in chapter 5. Briefly, it is difficult if not impossible for most people to permanently reduce their energy intake enough to lose a substantial amount of weight. This difficulty is compounded by the fact that dieting triggers a reflexive reduction in energy expenditure. As you voluntarily cut down on food intake, your efforts may be undone by an involuntary reduction in energy output.

The general failure of weight-reducing diets suggests that if you are ever going to achieve weight loss, you will have to increase energy output. An increase in energy output can be in addition to or instead of a decrease in energy intake. In either case, for this procedure to have permanent effects, it has to be a permanent change. Temporary changes produce only temporary results. This, of course, is the source of despair for the overnight-diet-success stories. Permanent weight loss following a temporary change in input or output only occurs in fairy tales and advertisements.

There are sound reasons why exercise can be recommended to most people. One simple, yet very important reason is that exercise can be fun. It is by no means always or necessarily fun, but certain types of exercise are often quite enjoyable. In contrast, dieting is never fun. It is not a matter of diets rarely being fun or not being much fun—diets are a miserable form of privation. Anyone who claims to enjoy dieting is either trying to sell you something or has a closetful of hair shirts.

Another reason to recommend exercise is that exercise is less likely to be harmful than dieting. That is not to say that exercise is without risks. Bruises, abrasions, bumps, and soreness are the stuff on which exercise is founded. There is a prevalent belief that if it doesn't hurt, it can't be very good for you. This self-punitive attitude toward exercise is almost certainly wrong, but the damage caused by it is usually not great. The antiexercise brigade delights in stories of people dropping dead while jogging or being run over by cars or being mugged. This is not good evidence in support of their eschewing exercise.

Closer examination of the cases of death following jogging has revealed a consistent pattern. The deaths almost always occur in those who have clear histories of heart problems and who ignore early warning signs that they may be overdoing it. Overexercise, much like overweight, can be dangerous, particularly for those who have heart disease. Neither condition (overexercise or overweight) is necessarily a particular health liability in itself.

It should also be remembered that a lot of people drop dead in just about every human endeavor each year. To isolate the relatively small number of deaths following exercise is deceptive and misleading. A jogger is no more liable to being mugged or run over than is any other pedestrian. In fact, since they are likely to be more nimble, joggers may enjoy a modest degree of immunity from these contemporary urban hazards.

Exercise is also clearly preferable to dieting in terms of its effects on your self-esteem. Exercise is a rather personally neutral pursuit in that if you do not reach your goal, you are not held to be particularly weak or vile. Dropping out of an exercise program causes little comment outside the circle of liniment fascists. The failure to achieve a burnished, lust-provoking physique is not widely considered to be a serious failure. It is merely not a positive achievement. Contrast this with the typical attitude toward failed dieters.

Fat people are seen as wilfully perpetrating their moral-aesthetic assault on the rest of us. Couple this with the enormous health bill that we are told we bear for their wanton excess, and you have a formidable indictment of fatness. Of course this is all vicious nonsense, but a large segment of the public either implicitly or explicitly subscribes to many of these views.

Fat people are held in low general esteem. An inevitable consequence of this is that many fat people come to loathe themselves. Their low sense of self-esteem is exacerbated by failed attempts at dieting. And fail they will. The probability of anyone succeeding at a diet is very low, but for those who really need to lose weight the probability of success is even lower. All of this exacts a frightful toll in terms of stress and unhappiness. The fat person who chooses to exercise instead of diet avoids a substantial portion of this needless harassment. This is a definite plus for exercise.

The Energy Value of Exercise

Before describing the role of exercise in weight reduction, it is necessary to differentiate between two types of exercise. These differences themselves have been sufficiently misunderstood to fuel a number of exercise myths. Most of the energy we use during typical sustained exercise, such as jogging, is derived from fatty acids. The fatty acids require oxygen for their combustion, hence the term *aerobic metabolism*.

The fact that aerobic exercise is totally oxygen dependent is a bit of a red herring. What is important about this type of exercise is that it uses fat for fuel and that its effects are widespread throughout the body. Aerobic activity mobilizes a large variety of physiological processes. This sort of exercise is held to be particularly good for the cardiovascular system.

The physiology and consequences of short-duration exertion are very different from those of aerobic activity. Intense short-term exertion is fueled almost entirely by the muscles' own reserves of glycogen. Glycogen use does not necessarily require oxygen, hence the term *anaerobic*. The reason why anaerobic metabolism is of very little overall importance in our physiology is that it is a relatively inefficient way to produce energy. Aerobic metabolism is about eight times more energetically efficient. Consequently, anaerobic metabolism is something of a short-term and emergency metabolic pathway. The anaerobic metabolism of glycogen fuels the muscular contractions that occur after death.

The effects of anaerobic exercise are limited to a relatively small group of muscles. On the other hand, aerobic exercise is assumed to have widespread systemic effects. The validity of this assumption will be discussed on page 151. Anaerobic exercise is best characterized as muscle building. One of the things that either form of physical training does is to increase the muscles' ability to store glycogen.

The idea of losing weight and increasing your general fitness at the same time is certainly an attractive one. Whether this is feasible or is just another pipe dream depends on how much one can reasonably increase energy expenditure through exercise. This question turns out to be far more complex than is generally appreciated. In order to place the question in its proper perspective, we will first present the simple gospel of the exercise advocates.

Some of the slenderness-through-exercise advocates claim that excess weight could be eliminated simply by increasing our daily energy expenditure by 50 percent. They present this sort of increase in energy expenditure as being merely a transition from slothfulness to liveliness. In terms of changing energy balance, this would be the equivalent of reducing energy intake by about one-third. The full efficacy of increasing energy expenditure by 50 percent depends on your concurrent energy intake remaining constant. Any reduction in energy intake during an exercise regimen would, of course, enhance the weight loss. The negative energy balance brought about by a 50 percent increase in daily energy expenditure would undoubtedly have a pronounced slenderizing effect.

The weight loss that would be produced by the above, rather idealized exercise regimen can be idealistically calculated as follows: Given a total daily energy expenditure of 2,600 kcal, a 50 percent increase (that is, 1,300 kcal) would mean that you would have to use 1,300 kcal of you to make up the difference. Hopefully, the part of you that would be used would be fat and not protein. A slight note of desperation enters this discussion when you realize that the energy value of fat is 4,000 kcal/lb. In other words, this program of sweating and groaning would require over three days to lose each lb of fat.

The more optimistic aspirants to weight loss would not be daunted by this rather low apparent level of payoff for their exercise program. After all, ten weeks equals 20 lb, twenty weeks equals 40 lb, and so on. On with the liniment and off with the weight! However, there is a potential fly in the liniment of this argument. Is it a reasonable expectancy for someone to be able to increase their overall energy output by 50 percent? Would this sort of increase in energy expenditure represent a transition from slothfulness to liveliness? Certainly, a number of experts have suggested the desirability of increases in energy expenditure of this order. But how much exercise would you have to do achieve this end? How much energy does exercise cost and just how much energy can anyone be expected to expend? The answers to these questions, to a large extent, determine the practicality of the exercise prescription. We will see, below, that it is not a very practical prescription for weight loss.

By exploring the upper limits of human energy expenditure we can more fully appreciate what the reasonable expectancy should be. One of the most fascinating studies of this sort was of a coal miner in the days before mining became heavily automated. The miner, who is known only as Jock E, was a strapping (5 feet 8 inches, 161 pounds) twenty-seven-year-old.

Jock's energy expenditure was calculated by the classic energy-balance procedure. This requires precise measurements of the energy value of what goes in (food), what comes out (urine and feces), and any change in weight. This procedure, while extremely tedious, can be very accurate. Unfortunately, because it is so labor intensive, it is not suitable for large-scale studies. In fact, this sort of study is rarely done anymore.

Jock's duties consisted mainly of hewing coal with a pickax and loading it into carts. He did this for sixty hours a week. By all counts his energy expenditure must have been very close to the upper limits of even very fit young men. Jock's average daily energy expenditure due to work was 1,800 kcal! This figure obviously far exceeds that attainable by at least 99 percent of those who attempt to lose weight through exercise. For our purposes it can be considered to represent an upper limit of energy expenditure.

It is useful to convert Jock's herculean level of energy expenditure to potential fat loss. Of course, like any sensible laborer, Jock ate enough so that he did not lose weight. However, if Jock had not increased his food intake to compensate for his work load, he would have lost about 3 lb of fat a week. This is the absolute maximum rate of fat loss that can be produced by extreme physical exertion during a sixty-hour work week. If Jock had starved himself in addition to working so hard, his theoretical weight loss might have been doubled. Fortunately, few people are so desperate and silly that they would combine extreme exercise with starvation. It would be very unhealthy, even dangerous. Very few fat people have anything like the time or physical fitness, to say nothing of the maniacal level of dedication, required to expend more than a small fraction of the energy that Jock did.

What about all of those tables that tell you things like a cup of coffee with one sugar and milk equals eighteen minutes of brisk walking, a piece of chocolate cake equals forty-five minutes of jogging, and so forth? These estimates of the exercise equivalents of various food are almost always based upon a glaringly incorrect assumption. As a result, they are wildly optimistic. These tables present the gross cost of exercise. They assume that the alternative to the exercise is virtually being in a coma. When we are not exercising, we are far from comatose. This is the key to understanding why exercise is not a very good way to lose weight.

Even if you are simply sitting in an armchair, you still expend a considerable amount of energy. This energy is used to maintain posture and for the movements of your torso, head, and limbs, This means that even while sitting quietly, you use much more energy than the reference value used typically in calculating the energy equivalents of exercise. The only meaningful energy cost of exercise is based upon the net value of the exercise. The net energy cost of exercise is the difference between resting-energy expenditure and the gross energy cost of the exercise. This figure paints a much less optimistic picture of the use of exercise in weight reduction than does the more commonly used gross energy value.

Expressed in these more realistic terms, exercise takes on a rather different luster. In order to use one pound of fat, you would have to play 100 holes of golf or 20 sets of tennis or scale the Eiffel Tower 12 times. In fact, the opponents of exercise could paint a still more dismal picture of exercise as an instrument of weight loss. The net value of exercise should really be expressed as the gross value less what you would have done if you had not gone jogging. When you are not exercising, you are probably not lying down immobile. If you did not jog, you might well have puttered about in the garden or visited the neighbors. These prosaic activities use much more energy than does the resting state. Taking them into account would still further diminish the net cost of exercise.

Exercise and Energy Balance

There are some other factors that tend to reduce the overall impact of exercise on body weight. For example, after exercise (particularly strenuous exercise), you are likely to rest. The more strenuous the exercise, the more complete the rest. The postexercise collapse could well reduce your energy expenditure to levels substantially lower than those you would have had if you had not exercised at all. Similarly, some types of exercise are very likely to produce a compensatory increase in food intake. This would, of course, substantially undo the aim of achieving a state of negative energy balance so that you can lose weight.

Alterations in food intake following exercise have been widely reported, yet their direction is still controversial. Some investigators have reported that exercise increases food intake, whereas others have reported decreases of similar magnitude. This is clearly an important issue to resolve, since changes in food intake could either amplify or totally negate any weight loss produced by exercise. It could well be that the nature of the diet before and during exercise is crucial in determining whether exercise increases or decreases food intake. This does not appear to have been systematically investigated.

There is still another way in which the effects of exercise on weight may be blunted. One of the major effects of training is to increase muscular efficiency. Any well-practiced act can be performed with less effort than the same act at an earlier stage of practice. This means, for example, that the more frequently you jog, the less energy you expend for a given amount of jogging. Training increases the amount of energy that goes into work and decreases the amount that is wasted as heat. This means that over time you must exercise more to achieve the same amount of energy expenditure.

The above considerations suggest that exercise is not nearly as good for losing weight as its more ardent proponents would have us believe; however, they do not in any way detract from the potential benefits of exercise for one's general health and well-being. There are even a couple of ways in which exercise could be substantially better for weight loss than the foregoing analysis would suggest. For instance, the net energy cost of exercise could be greatly increased if the increased energy expenditure produced during the exercise persisted afterward. If this were the case, even if you collapsed after your exertion, you would continue to expend more energy than normal. This is the ideal situation of apparently getting something for nothing—"just sit there and watch your fat melt away."

Alas, the postexercise elevation of energy expenditure is far from being an established fact. The most commonly cited evidence for this attractive phenomenon is a study of American college football players conducted in the 1930s. After a game, the football players showed an increase in energy expenditure that persisted for at least twenty-four hours. It should be pointed out that the evidence for increased energy expenditure was entirely indirect. An increase in energy expenditure was inferred from the fact that on the day after the game, the players' large food intake was not reflected in an appropriate weight gain.

A number of subsequent investigators have not been able to show the postulated exercise "echo effect" in either direct or indirect measures of energy expenditure. These negative findings could be taken to indicate that the postulated phenomenon did not exist. Alternately, and more optimistically, they could indicate the operation of variables that were not made explicit in the experiments. For example, it is possible that such an effect could be associated with a particular type of diet or exercise regimen or the state of fitness of the subjects. If this speculation is correct and the echo effect is real, whoever finds the key variables will have his or her name in lights.

Apart from the rather equivocal echo effect described above, there is another way in which the real cost of exercise could be greater than skeptics have suggested. In chapter 3 we discussed the thermic effect of food. This phenomenon, which is most often called diet-induced thermogenesis, is an important way of wasting energy. A proportion of the energy is all foods is converted to heat and radiated into the environment. If the proportion of energy wasted were increased, we would be in the enviable position of having our cake without its appearing around the waistline.

There have been suggestions that exercise increases diet-induced thermogenesis. Unfortunately, like so much of the lore of fatness and fitness, this issue has been sold to the public with a considerable degree of wishful thinking and no solid evidence. It would be lovely if exercise really did enhance diet-induced thermogenesis, but the existing data are not very persuasive. Advocates of the grunt and groan have been less than candid in their presentation of the case for this phenomenon.

The truth is that exercise appears to reduce, not increase, diet-induced thermogenesis in both rats and humans. Further, the more fit the subject, the greater is the reduction in thermogenesis. In response to a liquid meal of about 800 kcal (or roughly one-third their normal total daily energy intake) healthy, normal women increased their energy expenditure by about 22 percent. Essentially all of this energy was wasted. In marked contrast, female athletes only increased their energy expenditure by 10 percent in response to the same liquid meal. The extensively trained athletes wasted less than half as much of the energy as the control subjects.

These findings are exactly the reverse of what the apostles of exercise would want. Not only does exercise not add much to your voluntary energy expenditure, but it may actually reduce your involuntary energy expenditure. The more you train, the more pronounced the effect is. Much of the reason for the increased energetic efficiency following exercise is that exercise produces a fundamental shift in the way energy is stored.

Well-trained athletes owe much of their increased performance capability to the fact that they have great reserves of muscle glycogen. In contrast, nontrained people tend to store more of their energy intake as fat. This difference is important because producing fat is a far more energetically wasteful process than producing glycogen. This rather straightforward biochemical wisdom has some important implications that seem to have gone unnoticed.

In order to become fat, you must synthesize fat. However, synthesizing fat is a rather energetically wasteful process. A fat person requires a great deal of energy intake (that is, food) in order to add another pound of fat. A thin person requires much less food intake to add another pound of muscle. This means that, to a certain extent, fattening is a self-limiting process. Conversely, slimming is too. The evolutionary sense in this sort of arrangement should be obvious.

Nature does its best to avoid extremes of fatness or slimness. To enforce this evolutionary wisdom, we have developed physiological regulatory mechanisms that automatically alter our energetic efficiency. We can waste excess energy intake by radiating it as heat through thermogenesis. Additionally or alternatively, we can waste energy by building fat. The converse of these energy-wastage processes comes into play in times of energy shortage.

The message in this is that our level of fatness or slenderness is not simply the incidental outcome of how much we eat and/or exercise. Body weight is a rigorously defended physiological parameter. The physiological and biochemical mechanisms that defend our body weight have developed over millions of years and they will not be defeated easily by dieting. This should have become abundantly clear in the previous chapter, on dieting. It should be clear now that exercise may be an even less effective (if less harmful) means of losing weight than dieting.

The question "Is exercise a good way to lose weight?" appears to be rarely asked. This is perhaps because the exercise proponents simply assume that the answer is yes, whereas the exercise opponents don't care. If you are dogmatically antiexercise, you are not likely to be particularly concerned about your weight. On the other hand, if you are a true believer in exercise, you are not likely to be too concerned about the nature of the evidence you use to support your cause.

The core claims of the exercise brigade are that exercise facilitates weight loss and that it selectively promotes the loss of fat while sparing the muscle wastage that is common to diets. There are a few studies that in one way or another, could be seen as providing support for these claims. However, for each of these supporting studies there is probably a half dozen that show no such effects. Further, the positive studies share a common "informality," whereas the negative studies appear to be more rigorous.

This is one of those areas in which there is quite close agreement between theoretical predictions and reality. Theoretical and empirical considerations concur in suggesting that exercise is of little or no benefit in facilitating weight loss. Like it or not, this is what the data say. This does not in any way constitute an overall indictment of exercise; it merely indicates that weight loss is one sphere in which it has been oversold. The glorious allegations as to the miraculous benefits of exercise for weight loss are ill founded.

Shaping Your Body with Exercise

Even if you can swallow the bitter pill that exercise is not a good way to lose weight overall, you might still like to hang on to the notion that exercise is good for trimming selective fat deposits. A great many people want to improve their figures by shedding a little fat here and there. This demand has, of course, been met with a product. There is a booming business in "body sculpture." Advocates of this exercise variant have developed exercises that selectively target every flaccid fold, ridge, and valley of the body. If you have a fat stomach, droopy bottom, saggy neck, or bags under your eyes, there is an exercise or combination or exercises that will solve your problem. These are flogged aggressively in the mass media. Body sculpture has become big business.

The idea of trimming your fat belly with a program of sit-ups has been with us for a long time. The body-sculpture approach is merely an extension of this same logic to other regions of the body. However, there is something fundamentally wrong with it. It appears to have escaped general attention that sit-ups have never flattened a bulging belly. Given this inescapable fact, targeting other regions of the body for "spot reduction" appears doubly absurd. Sit-ups use stomach muscles to a far greater extent than is their usual lot. This exercise increases the glycogen-retaining ability of the muscles and develops new connective tissue. Sit-ups build stomach muscle. If you have a fat stomach and sit up religiously each day, eventually you will develop rippling, taut stomach muscles—crowned by the same flab you had before!

During sit-ups the stomach muscles do not get the message that they are supposed to draw their fuel from the nearby fat. They don't get the message because there is no way for them to get such a message. There is no system that tells any muscle where to draw its energy from. The energy used for sit-ups or for any other exercise is simply drawn from your general energy reserves—fat. If your only significant fat depot were your stomach, then the negative energy balance that might be produced by the exercise would probably reduce that fat mass.

What the body sculptors ignore is the fact that in the vast majority of people, fat is distributed relatively uniformly about the body. Consequently, when fat is used, it is drawn fairly uniformly from these widely spread reserves. Exercise can selectively target certain muscle groups, but it cannot selectively target particular far deposits.

Fat and muscle are entirely different tissues, each with its own distinct physiology. Further, unless you achieve a reasonably prolonged state of negative energy balance, no fat will be used at all. There are even data showing that very intense, short bursts of exercise tend to increase body weight. Weight lifters have used this principle for years.

The futility of the entire body-sculpting approach was recently demonstrated in professional tennis players. If anyone gets the opportunity to purge the fat from one arm, it is a tennis professional. One could say that every day they are sculpting their racquet arm. Consequently, their racquet arm should be less fat than their other arm. Careful measurements showed that these athletes have more muscle and even more bone in their racquet arm. However, there is no difference in the amount of fat in their two arms. Exercise is great for building muscles, but it is not very good for either local or general weight loss.

What Is Exercise Good For?

The previous section could be misconstrued as support for the antiathletic supporters. It is not. Instead, it is simply a step toward placing exercise in its proper perspective. The jockstrap fanatics have made claims for exercise that are as absurd as those made for diets by the sleaziest charlatans ever to hire a tent. As a result of the messianic delusions of the Adidas set, a sizable sector of the public has been turned off something that may well be very good for them. Who wants to be associated with a bandwagon populated by such drooling crazies? The contagion from absurd and harmful ideas permeates the entire health, body-weight, nutrition, and fitness business. There is so much rampant silliness that many people have developed a general skepticism toward everything to do with any of these areas. This is unfortunate and unhealthy.

It is helpful to take a look at the value of exercise from an evolutionary perspective. Ritualized exercise such as games and sports have, until very recent times, been only an insignificantly small proportion of total human energy expenditure. It does not make much sense that suddenly frenetic devotion to these sweaty pursuits should be of such lifesaving value. It is not impossible, just not very likely. There is no precedent for this sort of instant evolution in the history of our species. That a minority pastime would become the salvation of our species virtually overnight is a physiological fairy tale.

Exercise may turn out to be a bit like weight loss in that it is very good for a significant minority. Also like weight loss, exercise is not the public health imperative it is widely made out to be. This parallel is reinforced by considering the groups who can most clearly benefit from exercise. As was the case with weight loss, the groups most likely to benefit from exercise are those who have diabetes or high blood pressure. However, in marked contrast to weight loss, exercise is a reasonably attainable goal for these people. Substantially improving one's physical fitness is possible for almost anyone. On the other hand, losing a substantial amount of weight is possible for almost no one. Further, even if the exercise does not do much good, it is not likely to do much harm.

We can better understand the real benefits of exercise by more closely considering the purpose for which it was originally developed. Exercise is first and foremost physical training. The object of physical training is to improve performance on some athletic task. Exercise is indispensable in this context. Without constant training, it is impossible to be a first-rate athlete.

The almost universal assumption that physical fitness is a sign of good health is largely unsubstantiated. It is clear that being unfit is often associated with being unhealthy. It is far less clear whether being particularly fit is associated with being particularly healthy. Beyond a modest level of fitness, further improvements certainly improve athletic performance, but it is far less certain that these have corresponding benefits for health.

This argument raises the hackles of the exercise advocates. It is considered little short of treasonous in many circles. Criticizing, or even failing to extol, the universal virtues of exercise is held to be tantamount to aiding and abetting moral turpitude. Some see it as a frank advocation of the corruption of our precious bodily fluids. When the forces of natural patriotism hear of this heresy, they will be tightening the laces on their combat sneakers and heading in my direction. But the truth stands by itself. I had nothing to do with its making.

What about the data showing that activity protects men against coronary heart disease? This protection by itself should be enough to secure a place for exercise in preventive medicine. For example, a survey of about eighteen thousand middle-aged male public servants showed that the most active men had much lower rates of mortality from all causes and cardiovascular disease in particular. This result remained even when the effects of smoking were statistically calculated (see chapter 2 for a discussion of multivariate statistics).

The obvious problem raised by findings such as these is determining whether the men lived longer because they were more active, or whether they were more active because they were healthier in the first place. If the latter were the case, then the differences in life expectancy would simply reflect initial health differences, and being more active would simply be a marker of this good health.

In order to make valid long-term comparisons between groups, the groups must be reasonably equivalent in the first place. Epidemiological data are often very inadequate in this respect. To use such data to support a health-facilitating function of exercise is not justified. At best, epidemiological data are mildly suggestive that exercise may provide some degree of protection from certain health hazards.

There is nothing wrong with suggestive data as such. They may be quite useful as part of a larger argument in which there are a number of independent lines of evidence pointing to the same conclusion. As yet, the overall structure supporting the general health benefits of exercise is not very substantial. The entire argument is essentially suggestive. Exercise may well improve the cardiovascular health of middle-aged men, and that is a valuable result. It is, however, a very long way from showing that exercise is the great health discovery of the late twentieth century.

Some of the epidemiological data that are used to support the claims for the general health benefits of exercise may be turned to quite different purposes. For example, a comparison among groups of men from the American cities of Framingham, Massachusetts; San Juan, Puerto Rico; and Honolulu, Hawaii, is interpreted as indicating that the men who exercise most had the lowest cardiovascular mortality. In fact in that study, exercise was not measured at all. The safest group reported themselves as eating more than the other group, but they did not weigh any more. The experimenter then inferred that the safe group must have exercised more!

Of course, any rational consideration of the nature of energy balance (see chapter 4) and exercise (present chapter) indicates that their reasoning is grossly wrong. If their basic data are correct, it is a certainty that the safe group had a higher energy expenditure. However, whether this difference was due to exercise or something else is another question entirely. It should come as no great surprise that these data do not appear to have been used to support the position that overeating protects against heart disease.

In fact, there are data which flatly contradict the optimistic views on the benefits of exercise for cardiovascular health. These data come from a study involving several hundred men who underwent an intensive twelve-week physical fitness course. These men received thorough medical examinations both before and after the program, as well as four to six years later. In terms of a number of coronary "risk factors," the program produced no short-term or long-term benefits.

These discordant data notwithstanding, the value of exercise in maintaining cardiovascular health in middle-aged men is becoming increasingly apparent. The precise mechanism for the preventive effect of exercise is not clear, but it is probably not through any general strengthening of the heart.

The popular idea that aerobic exercise strengthens the heart is not supported by much evidence. The strengthening produced by aerobic or anaerobic exercise tends to be confined to the skeletal muscles directly used in the exercise. Heart muscle is not skeletal muscle and is not directly involved in the exercise. The heart and lungs may not be subject to anything like the training effects seen in limb muscles such as those of the legs and arms. This has been vividly demonstrated by giving people aerobic exercise in which the person can only use one limb.

One-limb aerobic exercise can be done on an exercise bicycle. It simply requires that during the first stage of the training the person uses only one leg to pedal. If the exercise produced a general improvement in heart and lung performance, these people would have a substantial head start when the previously unused leg began its training in the second stage of the experiment. No such systemic improvements were seen at the start of the second stage. The unused leg had to be trained from scratch. It did not reap the aerobic benefits that should have accrued from the training of the first leg. It looks very much as if the effects of the aerobic training were almost entirely restricted to those leg muscles directly used in the exercise.

I have gradually moved toward the position that exercise may have some benefits for cardiovascular health, if only for middle-aged men. We will see below that exercise may also be very good for anyone with diabetes or high blood pressure. The question is, since exercise does not appear to strengthen the heart, how does it exert its beneficial effects on health?

Exercise and Blood Chemistry

There is another important and intriguing way in which exercise could improve cardiovascular health without improving overall cardiovascular functioning. This other way is through a variety of effects on blood chemistry.

A great many heart problems are actually secondary to vascular problems. For example, high blood pressure is an obvious culprit in all sorts of lethal heart problems. High blood pressure is generally due to problems in the vasculature outside of the heart. In turn, many vascular problems are due to abnormalities in blood lipids, such as cholesterol. High blood pressure and high blood cholesterol levels have clear and undisputed implications for cardiovascular function. Either of these conditions is a danger sign, and the combination is frightening.

There is an increasing body of evidence showing that exercise may exert much of its beneficial effects on the cardiovascular system by altering the way lipids are handled in the blood. This indirect mode of action is very different from the direct heart-strengthening route that has been the traditional favorite of exercise advocates. In particular, exercise may increase the ratio of high-density lipoprotein (HDL) to low-density lipoprotein (LDL). HDLs are lipid scavengers and LDLs are lipid depositers. Thus, increasing the ratio of HDLs to LDLs would favor the scavenging of lipids from the arteries. This would tend to make the development of atherosclerosis less likely. A high ratio of HDLs to LDLs is nature's own medicine for atherosclerosis. Anything that enhances HDLs and/or inhibits LDLs is likely to be good medicine for anyone with lipid problems.

There is a good deal of evidence that HDLs are enhanced by exercise. However, it is still unclear as to how much exercise is required to produce the effect. One of the early reports suggested that it required at least fifteen miles of jogging per week to produce a noticeable effect. An even more pessimistic report suggested that at least thirty-five miles of weekly jogging was required. The latter figure is beyond the reasonable limits of any but those who sleep in track suits.

The beneficial effects of exercise on blood lipids were first applied on a large scale in Finland. Finnish men are notorious in the cardiovascular trade for their extremely high incidence of heart attacks. These data are interesting in that they concern a sample drawn at random from the general community. Most of the other data on this subject are more difficult to interpret since they are based upon people who are more or less exercise devotees. Further, in some of the other groups the runners had unusually low meat intake, which by itself will tend to increase the ratio of HDLs to LDLs.

A four-month program of mainly aerobic exercises produced substantial increases in the crucial ratio of HDLs to LDLs in Finnish men. Further, the runners in the sample had no initial advantage over the nonrunners. The latter finding suggests that the results described above were not simply artifacts of starting with a biased sample.

Note that even the data from this Finnish experiment are still a long way from endorsing the position that exercise is the cure for the health woes of our species. They merely suggest that exercise may tilt the balance of HDLs to LDLs in such a way as to favor more efficient scavenging of blood lipids. It is possible that these effects are restricted to middle-aged men, but it is more likely that they have broader application.

To a large extent, this same end may be achieved by dietary means. A reduction in dietary intake of fats, particularly saturated fats, accompanied by an increase in carbohydrates, will achieve similar results without having to sweat. It should not be forgotten that many people do not have problems with their lipids in the first place. If you have an adequate ratio of HDLs to LDLs and reasonable levels of blood lipids, it is unlikely that exercise will do much for your cardiovascular health.

Exercise also has some important benefits to offer diabetics. Diabetes is a condition of high insulin levels accompanied by low insulin sensitivity. The resultant failure to maintain blood glucose levels within safe limits plays havoc with small blood vessels all over the body. Among those organs that are most likely to suffer damage are the heart, brain, and eyes. Diabetes is a killer disease.

Insulin sensitivity may be increased by weight reduction. Why this occurs is not well understood very well, but there is little doubt that diabetics are among those who can genuinely profit from weight loss. However, there are also abundant data that show that diabetics may have even more difficulty than nondiabetics in losing weight. As desirable as weight loss may be for them, very few diabetics can lose much weight. Further, even fewer diabetics can maintain weight loss for a significant length of time.

On the other hand, many diabetics show greatly improved insulin sensitivity simply as a result of exercise. In marked contrast to weight loss, exercise is an attainable goal for most diabetics. Unfortunately, many fat diabetics are so obsessed with a futile battle against their fat that they ignore this real therapeutic alternative.

Exercise also appears to be good medicine for those with high blood pressure. This was forcefully demonstrated in a group of fat, hypertensive Swedish women. Following a six-month exercise course, these women all showed substantial reductions in blood pressure. This demonstration is particularly persuasive since few of the women lost weight. These data also point to an association between the beneficial effects of exercise for diabetics and hypertensives because the largest reductions in blood pressure were seen in the women who initially had high insulin levels.

Overall, the present analysis indicates that there is a definite role for exercise in promoting good health. In contrast, there is little, if any, role for exercise in weight reduction. Exercise may be of real value in conditions such as atherosclerosis, diabetes, and hypertension. It may even slow the bone deterioration that occurs in some old people. However, for most people exercise probably has little to offer besides bigger muscles.

Devotees of the grunt and groan have been seriously misleading the general public. Exercising has only a fraction of the miraculous power that they claim it has. Exercise might be a great hobby, but it will not save us from either moral or physical decay. At best, it may slightly delay one form of decay and marginally enhance the enjoyment of the other. In defense of exercise, it should be added that, unlike diet madness, exercise mania is relatively harmless.

CHAPTER 7

FIGHTING FAT WITH EVERYTHING ELSE

When diets fail repeatedly (as they almost always do), some dieters try to get a new lever on their fatness by undergoing psychotherapy. The psychotherapist can take one of two courses with weight problems. One is to help the patient to learn to live with his or her current weight and forget about trying to lose it. This course is rarely taken except in the case of anorexia nervosa, when the patient is already too thin. This is rather unfortunate, since most fat people will ultimately have to learn to make this adjustment. Such "live with it" counseling could well be of real value to many fat people, but they are not likely to get it from a psychotherapist.

The other and by far the most frequent course taken by psychotherapists is to focus on curing the patient's eating problems. Patients are made to record the exact circumstances under which they eat and the details of what they eat and sometimes even the number of bites and chews they make. The logic behind this is that if you show patients why they overeat, they will see the folly of their ways and repent by eating normally. Therapists with a Freudian orientation may try to discover the roots of the patient's oral tendencies. More eclectic therapists simply try to extirpate excessive eating, often using guilt as a bludgeon.

In the final analysis psychotherapy is of little benefit to fat people. This could only be expected, since fat people rarely have an eating pathology to rectify. It is not a bad bet that more than a few fat people have come away from psychotherapists with eating problems that they did not have in the first place.

Psychotherapy

It is now beyond doubt that relatively few fat people actually overeat. This is not deny the possibility that at some time in their lives fat people may have been overeaters. That possibility is pretty much impossible to prove or disprove. In either case, the lack of a current eating problem suggests that the therapist does not have a valid target to attack. The singular lack of success of psychotherapists with fat people supports this contention. The psyche of some fat people may well be twisted, but it is likely to be the result of the stigma of fatness. Psychological problems probably cause very little fatness, but fatness undoubtedly causes many psychological problems.

A slightly more enlightened approach focuses entirely on overt behavior and ignores the hypothetical psychodynamic processes that lurk beneath the surface. Behavior modification is often used as an adjunct to more traditional forms of psychotherapy. When behavior modification therapy tries to eliminate overeating, its likelihood of helping fat people is little better than that of the conventional psychotherapies. This is because few fat people are overeaters, and you cannot correct a nonexistent pathology. However, the relative enlightenment of this approach involves trying to restructure eating behavior in order to adapt the dieter to the life of privation that is necessary to maintaining weight loss.

The vast majority of fat people are like alcoholics in that, in order to maintain any therapeutic improvement, they must become permanently abstemious. When dieters "fall off the wagon," even if their lapse only involves eating normally, they are very likely to get fat again. The popular idea of shedding some weight with a "crash" diet and then resuming normal eating, works in only a minuscule proportion of dieters.

In spite of the clear worthlessness of crash diets, the vast majority of diet merchants either implicitly or explicitly suggest that their diet is only a temporary inconvenience. Temporary diets almost never produce more than temporary results. Most successful long-term weight losers are committed to a life-long fast. This sort of ascetic dedication is possible, but few people are willing or able to achieve it.

This decidedly pessimistic scenario applies primarily to people who have a lot of weight to lose. If you only have a small amount of weight to lose, the picture is rather brighter. Minor weight adjustments may not mobilize the metabolic machinery that so effectively combats attempts to lose larger amounts of weight (see chapter 4). Unfortunately, once weight gets into the range where it is a genuine health hazard, it is likely to be defended by metabolic compensation and consequently becomes very difficult to change.

The importance of small weight losses that are not related to health should not be trivialized. For many people such minor cosmetic adjustments in weight are of immense psychological importance. For the affluent and fashion conscious an extra ten pounds can mean the difference between retaining and discarding an entire wardrobe. Ten pounds one way or the other will not in itself have any effect on the health of anyone, but it may still be of great personal significance.

Fortunately, minor weight adjustments do not require any wonder diets. For most people, reducing body weight by, say 5 percent, simply requires an appropriate reduction in food intake. Your likelihood of losing weight may also be increased (if only slightly) by exercise. It is really very simple. The easiest way to achieve the negative energy balance essential to weight loss is to decrease energy intake and to increase energy expenditure. This technique does not require professional, quasi-professional (professional charges without professional expertise), or amateur assistance. Small weight losses are an ideal do-it-yourself project. If you look at diets as experiments with your own physiology, you are on the right track. When diets become a test of your moral worth, you are in trouble.

Weight-Loss Groups

One drawback of psychotherapy is that it is expensive. The fact that psychotherapy is so ineffective in promoting weight loss makes it expensive, even if it were free. Not only that, but the solitary visit to the therapist is no longer very fashionable. We live in an age still writhing in the clutches of pan-Californianism. The word is togetherness. Don't hide your failure to lose weight, make it a shared experience!

In their abject desperation to lose weight, millions of Americans have fallen prey to an alien, totalitarian ideology that in any other country would be called "socialist" dieting. Fear of fat has succeeded in an arena where national budgets have failed. Perhaps it is a bit inaccurate to characterize the weight-loss-group approach as socialist dieting. It is really socialist only in that it has a large-scale community orientation. It is, in general, far too immersed in making money to be truly socialist. Although there are a few nonprofit weight-loss groups, for the most part they are big-time, big-money operations. The biggest of them all is Weight Watchers, with millions of paying customers worldwide. Weight Watchers is a division of Heinz Foods, and it contributes handsomely toward Heinz's healthy corporate balance sheet. The corporate colonels would certainly characterize this as yet another example of doing well by doing good.

The secret behind the incredible success of the commercial weight-loss organizations is motivation, structure, and marketing. It would not be too uncharitable to say that motivation and structure are secondary to marketing. Clearly, these groups offer something the public wants and they have not been hiding their light under a bushel.

The motivation offered by the diet-group approach resides in the fact that they are closely modeled on Alcoholics Anonymous. The idea is that by sharing your affliction with other understanding sufferers you establish a mutually supportive atmosphere. It is this support system that is likely to keep you on the wagon. There is no conceivable dieting problem that is not represented in a large group such as Weight Watchers. The moral is that you are not alone.

This system is enhanced by a very complete structure to guide your efforts toward slenderness. Diet groups provide menus to suit virtually every taste and, unlike many fad diets, their menus are usually nutritionally sound. The large number of these menus that are now available means that dieting does not have to be quite so boring as it has traditionally been. They save you the bother of having to plan interesting, nutritionally sound, yet low-energy meals. This is the heart of their structured approach.

The dietary structure is made even easier for you by the fact that groups such as Weight Watchers are thoughtful enough to provide the very products that you need to closely follow the chosen path. In addition, many of these groups have even discovered exercise. Weight Watchers' exercise routine is cutely named Pepstep. All in all, the weight-loss groups offer a true "womb to tomb" approach to weight loss. Join one of these groups and you may well never again be faced with the difficulty of having to think for yourself. You can rest assured that all of the correct decisions will be made in paneled boardrooms, by executives who have only your best interests at heart.

By this point the critical reader may have noticed that I have been avoiding the only important question one really has to ask. Does joining one of these weight-loss groups increase your likelihood of being a successful dieter? Here what should be a fairly simple answer becomes shrouded in mystery. Some of these groups point out that to provide statistics on their success rate is impossible, since as soon as their customers lose the desired amount of weight, they become ex-customers. Others say that such information is strictly confidential and to divulge it would be akin to violating the secrecy of the confessional.

Even a prominent American consumer group, in their rating of various diet schemes, gushes superlatives on the group approach. The peculiarity of this high praise is that it is made without even considering the fundamental issue of whether these groups actually help people to lose weight. Strangely, they actually do talk about success at some length, but it is about the commercial success of the organization!

The standard dodge taken when the thorny issue of results is raised is that these groups are good for some people. Of course they are, but so is virtually every diet hustle that has ever been flogged in the marketplace. A certain percentage of people will show improvements in almost any condition in response to almost any treatment or to no treatment at all. The question that any therapist of integrity must eventually deal with is, does his or her therapy produce better than chance or placebo results?

It is this vital question that pulls the plug on the diet groups. The fact that they so sedulously avoid a straight, sensible answer to the question should be tip-off enough. If they had real success to offer, they would be screeching figures on success rates from the rooftops. Independent evaluation of the success rates of various diet groups paints a much less rosy picture than they would like the public to see. Diets and exercise are not very effective ways of losing weight (see chapters 5 and 6). There is no reason to expect the group approach to suddenly turn these sow's ears into silk purses. They haven't.

When you can wheedle any data out of the diet groups, they are usually in the form "*X* percent of our customers have been in our program for two years or more have lost an average of *Y* pounds." This sort of figure not very skillfully avoids several important points. The first and least important point is that *Y* pounds is fairly meaningless if you do not know the original weight of the group. A more relevant figure would be weight loss as a percentage of original weight.

The false impression that raw (that is, not expressed as percentages) weight-loss figures may be illustrated as follows. One weight-loss center advertised that over a six-month period one of their groups lost an average of about 20 pounds. However, if the average initial weight of the group was 250 pounds, the fact that, after six months in the program, they still weighed about 230 pounds is hardly a great success.

More important is the fact that even when the diet groups do divulge a little data, they are always short-term success stories. The commercial weight-loss groups never give any indication of the long-term success of their customers. Even if the initial weight loss is very large, it is critical to know whether the eventual relapse rate is as bad as it is for all other treatments. Absolutely none of the commercial groups gives any figures at all about the relapse rates of their customers. There is therefore no reason at all to think that they have succeeded where all others have failed. To the contrary, their very silence tells the whole story.

Another important deficiency of typical group weight-loss success data is that they never reveal the dropout rate. This is a critical figure because it shows a much more realistic indication of the chances of success. Unfortunately, the dropout rate from diet groups is uniformly and extremely high. One major Australian weight-loss company was found to lose 98 percent of their customers within the first year! If even 50 percent of the remaining dieters lost a large amount of weight, they would still have an overall success rate of only 1 percent! Nobody could do business for long with such a low success rate if anyone found out about it.

The only way commercial weight-loss organizations can continue to do a roaring business while achieving such pathetic results is by obscuring their own failure. Alas, this is what weight-loss marketing is all about. Get their attention. Get them into the tent. Get them signed up on the dotted line and let the devil take the hindmost. All the rhetoric and marketing in the world do not add up to weight loss. They do, however, add up to good business. It is the community at large who is getting the business.

Pills and Potions

The major reason why neither diets nor exercise are very good ways to lose weight is that they require more willpower than most of us can provide. It is an immutable truth that if you diet and exercise long enough, you have to lose weight. The laws of physics cannot be beaten by anyone.

The problem is that invoking the laws of physics on your behalf requires a formidable amount of willpower. Similarly, if you maintain the negative energy balance that you achieved through dieting and/or exercising, you can lose as much weight as you like and maintain any weight loss forever. Initially invoking the desired laws of physics on your behalf is difficult, but the amount of willpower required to stay permanently thin would make Clark Kent blanch.

For this reason, many have succumbed to the lure of pills and potions. These preparations neatly sidestep the major diet hurdle of willpower. Why get a psychological hernia when you can get better by dropping a few pills? Pills and potions promise the dieter's Eldorado of slenderness with no more effort than it takes to swallow. They also nicely illustrate the two poles of dieting approaches: the rational if misguided on the one side and grasping lunacy on the other.

We already know that the negative energy balance essential to weight loss requires either a reduction in energy input or an increase in energy output. This provides a neat organization scheme for looking at the nature of diet pills. They are all essentially directed at either decreasing intake or increasing output.

One way to decrease intake is to fill your stomach. There are a number of nonnutritive "bulking" agents available. They sport a variety of names, ranging from the rather sinister chemical name methylcellulose to the appealingly natural product alfalfa. In either case the aim is exactly the same. They seek to induce satiety and thwart hunger by filling the void in your stomach that you would normally stuff with all sorts of fattening foods.

This whole logic is based upon erroneous assumptions. Stomach distension is rarely the signal that terminates eating, nor is stomach emptiness the cue which initiates eating. One of the most impressive features of both human and animal food intake is the ability to adjust intake to compensate for changes in the nutritional value of the food. If you dilute the energy value of food by 50 percent, rats and humans simply double intake to keep the overall energy input constant. Any species that could not make such a simple adjustment to changes in energy availability would have been extinct long ago.

Thus, theoretical considerations suggest that inert bulking agents should not be very effective in bringing about weight loss. They make about as much sense as trying to reduce intake by placing small meals behind a magnifying glass to trick you into thinking you are eating a large meal. Actually, an approximation of this silly suggestion is already in the marketplace. One popular diet suggests that you use small plates and cutlery!

It should come as no surprise that these age-old wonders are not really so wonderful at all. They didn't work way back when they were discovered and they don't work now. Even giving these old products a new "natural" name will not transmute this water into wine. Just the same, virtually every pharmacy and absolutely every health food shop in the Western world still offers an extensive range of this nonsense.

The nineteenth century left us another dietary legacy besides bulking agents. Like bulking agents this one also has that valuable "natural" ring to it. However, unlike bulking agents, this treatment works on the output end of the energy-balance equation. This second hangover from the last century is the range of thyroid preparations that is still being flogged all over the place.

The fact that the thyroid gland was in some way involved in regulating basal metabolism was known, if not at all understood, in the nineteenth century. It was thought that fat people got that way because of a chronically underactive thyroid gland. Consequently, there was great interest in developing and discovering agents that would enhance thyroid activity.

The likely futility of using thyroid preparations in the treatment of fat people is suggested by several considerations. One is that, while there are a few fat people with thyroid deficiencies, there are probably at least as many thin people with exactly the same thyroid deficiencies. The vast majority of fat people have nothing at all wrong with their thyroid. This, by itself, would tend to suggest that the thyroid is not the right tree to be barking up.

Not only that, but fat people do not, in general, have low basal metabolic rates. There is now a great deal of evidence showing that basal metabolism is quite closely related to body mass. Consequently, fat people have rather higher rates of basal metabolism because they have more body mass. Further, the only doses of thyroid preparations that do much to increase energy expenditure are generally toxic. A high enough dose of almost any poison will increase energy expenditure. To suggest that this is a valid option for losing weight is, of course, absurd.

One old dodge taken by the floggers of thyroid products is to use more exotic sources for their hormones. One merchant proudly and patriotically advertises that their hormone is exclusively from American, corn-fed (blond, blue-eyed?) hogs. None of your swarthy, foreign, garlic-tainted hormone for them. Others endow alligator thyroid with the magic that is so patently absent from more mundane thyroid preparations. Alas, whether it is from alligator, pig, or aardvark, it is all hogwash for weight loss.

The bottom line is that thyroid hormones are both rather dangerous and ineffective for producing weight loss. One source of their danger is that they tend to increase the rate of loss of lean body mass (that is, muscle). The purpose of a diet is to lose fat and not muscle. Thyroid hormones tend to promote the loss of muscle, not fat. For that reason alone, they are just what the dieter does not need.

Another potentially lethal side effect of thyroid preparations is that they may alter the contractile properties of heart muscle. Since many of those who most urgently need to lose weight already have some sort of cardiovascular problem, to give them anything that may exacerbate that problem is sheer madness. In fact, one potential therapeutic use of thyroid hormones is to lower serum lipids in patients who have atherosclerosis. However, this application was discontinued when the dangerous effects on heart muscle were discovered.

Quite apart from their dangerous side effects, thyroid hormones are just not very effective in facilitating weight loss. A number of controlled clinical trials illustrate this point. In one substantial group that used thyroid hormones in addition to dieting, the results after two years were dismal. Of two hundred very obese patients, twenty-four had maintained a weight loss of twenty pounds, twelve had kept losses of forty pounds, and only one of the two hundred was still at an ideal weight! Clearly, if this is how thyroid hormones help a diet, they do not need this kind of help.

The mainstay of the diet-pill industry has been and continues to be the appetite suppressant. Since fatness is seen as being due to overeating and overeating is due to being too hungry, the solution is obvious. Reduce appetite and body weight will follow. Catering to the immense demand for pills to defeat our own rapaciousness has become very big business for the drug companies. It is also a lucrative hunting ground for the quacks and charlatans who hover around diet carrion. There is a quite astonishing array of compounds that claim to be able to suppress your appetite. They range from the nuts, raisins, and herbs of the counterculture to the pharmacological heavy metal of the legitimate drug trade.

Appetite suppressants have a fairly short history, since it was not until very recently that any sane person wanted to curb his or her appetite. This history of the development of our antipathy for our own appetites for food is a grim chapter for humankind.

Like so many of the discoveries of modern pharmacology, the appetite-suppressing properties of drugs were an accident. Appetite has been suppressed since time immemorial by a depressing variety of diseases and toxins. Quite reasonably, loss of appetite continues to be a psychiatric symptom that is regarded with some gravity. Perhaps the first time anyone actually felt good at the same time that his or her appetite was inhibited was after chewing on the leaves of the coca plant.

Cocaine was a real discovery. It made you feel peppy, not hungry, and generally ready to take on the world. the Peruvian Indians gave the world cocaine. By all accounts they are still paying the price.

Cocaine is best characterized as nature's own amphetamine ("speed"). Amphetamine, being a laboratory chemical, has attracted far more fear and loathing than its South American relative, cocaine. The truth is, both in terms of what they do and how they do it, amphetamine and cocaine are nearly identical. Both of these substances are powerful appetite suppressants, most other appetite suppressants are essentially variations on the same theme.

There is a compelling argument for the case that the worldwide abuse of amphetamines, cocaine, and all of their relatives is directly due to the efforts of some of the major drug companies. Huge quantities of these compounds had been synthesized by both sides in World War II. During the war they became virtually a standard dietary supplement in times of combat. In this context they were used to reduce fatigue so that the troops could fight longer and harder. They were seen as a simple tool for increasing military productivity.

Much to the chagrin of the drug companies, the war ended just as the stockpiles of speed and its friends had reached record levels. A solution was quickly provided by the marketing departments. Given the fact that they had vast quantities of a product for which the public had no use, they had to create a use. It wasn't very difficult. These little red pills could help you get through the dreariness of the day and even shave off a little of that unwanted postwar buldge. Within two years of the end of the war, the world was in the throes of its first drug-abuse epidemic. People tended to blame it on the war. The corporate criminals escaped unscathed.

Amphetamines and their relatives are not harmless little pills. These drugs produce a strong physical and psychological dependence. They also produce a variety of alarming cardiovascular effects that can be dangerous or even fatal. Not only that, but in surprisingly small doses they produce a very close approximation of paranoid schizophrenia. Devotees of speed become suspicious and withdrawn. They often have delusions of all sorts of evil machinations directed specifically against them.

The paranoid delusions triggered by speed are at the source of a frightening array of crimes of violence. The cold-bloodedness and grizzliness of these crimes is legendary in police circles. Speed is very bad medicine.

Much of the effort of the drug companies has been directed toward developing variants of speed that share its appetite-suppressing results but not its other nasty properties. To a certain extent, this molecular juggling process has been successful. There are now numerous appetite suppressants that do not have anywhere near the abuse potential of their recent relatives, the amphetamines. These are still mostly prescription drugs, although some of the milder ones are available on demand in many countries. They continue to constitute a large source of income for a number of drug companies.

In spite of their widely publicized dangers, the demand for amphetamine-related "diet pills" continues to be strong. Government legislation around the world has greatly restricted the availability of the parent compounds. The deluge of antidrug legislation, which reached nearly hysterical levels in the 1970s, has had little effect other than to drive them underground. It has generated a vigorous and lucrative business in backyard chemistry.

The great pity of it all is that, in addition to having so many nasty side effects, the appetite suppressants just do not produce the desired effect of facilitating weight loss. They all produce an initial reduction in appetite, but this reduction steadily diminishes over time. Their small initial effect soon become no effect at all. All the dieter is left with is a handful of side effects.

To add insult to this pharmacological injury, when you stop taking appetite suppressants, there is usually a "rebound" effect. In the immediate postdrug period there is often an explosive increase in appetite. This is usually accompanied by a large and rapid increase in weight. Appetite suppressants often produce an overall increase in weight!

The myriad new products that appear each year may be more or less chemically novel, but the overall story is almost always exactly the same. They differ mainly in the side effects they produce, not in their effectiveness. None of them really works, so it becomes a matter of choosing the pill that causes you the least distress. One of the recent new hopes in this area was the drug fenfluramine. In terms of its mode of action it is quite different from the traditional amphetamine derivatives. Fenfluramine turns out to be no more effective in suppressing appetite, but it does have an unfortunate tendency to produce a severe depression when its use is stopped. If this is pharmacological progress, who needs it?

The blind faith in appetite suppressants as the answer to weight loss appears to be strongest in those who prescribe the pills and in those who have never taken them. This is indicated by a simple consumer survey of those who have dieted with and without the aid of pills. The verdict of the consumers is clear. They show a very strong preference for diets alone, without pills of any sort. If you are not going to lose weight, you might as well fail with a minimum of side effects.

The essential ethical integrity of the mainstream drug trade with respect to fatness stands in sharp contrast to the grab-and-run attitude of the peripheral pill and potion pushers. Here we encounter the same unfortunate recipe that riddles the whole fat business: Find a peg, fuel some fears, make lots of promises, get a fistful of money, and sprint to the bank.

The sheer numbers of quack diet pills and potions (I don't recall having seen any suppositories) makes it quite impossible to do them justice, or alas injustice, in a book of this length. Nonetheless, they share enough common features so that they may really be handled as a group. Perhaps their most striking common characteristic is their central aim of providing financial security for those who sell them. After this it is all window dressing.

Another essential ingredient of quack pharmacology is a liberal sprinkling of genuine or almost genuine scientific terminology. The megaconcept is the scientific buzzword. You read a scientific journal or the *Reader's Digest* interpretation thereof and find out what looks to be a hot new number. It should combine an element of novelty with a certain amount of familiarity. You don't want to frighten the public off by making them do any unnecessary thinking.

The essential flavor of the shopfront and mail-order pharmacologists can be captured by listing a few phrases from some of their recent literature:

- Would you like to lose weight while you sleep?
- Every beautiful body begins with amino acids.
- Arginine, ornithine—the fat burners!
- Japanese super pill guarantees rapid weight loss!
- Natural bio-active weight-loss compound . . .
- Virtually eliminates the need to diet!
- No more fat—no more cellulite—no more dieting!
- Eat all you want and still lose weight!
- The pill does all the work!
- Metabolism profile B—the key to weight loss . . .
- Chinese herbal formula destroys type III fat!
- Flushes calories right out of your body!

Not surprisingly, many products offer incontrovertible evidence of their effectiveness. Some of the alleged evidence is in the form of testimonials from people they tell you are famous personalities. I've never heard of any of them, but maybe I've led a sheltered life. Much of the remaining evidence consists of testimonials from converts who are even more unknown and untraceable.

Anyone who tries to validate these miracles is effectively blocked from the start, since the beneficiaries of the miracles are identified only by initials (Mrs J. K., from somewhere). Nor are the miracle merchants willing to release their names even to bona fide investigators. This type of vanish-when-you-try-to-grab-it characteristics has been euphemistically labeled shyness. The shyness phenomenon is an unmistakable hallmark of the bunco artist. The evidence the diet dream merchants offer as to the effectiveness of their products is either grossly inadequate or entirely nonexistent.

From time to time these hustlers even offer money-back guarantees. Consumer-protection agencies around the world are awash with the backlog of unsatisfied claims lodged against the fly-by-night diet pharmacologists. Strangely, even when the guarantees are genuine, many disheartened dieters don't try to claim on them. The merchants correctly read the essential defeatism they themselves help to grind into the dieting desperadoes.

There is one relatively new antifat potion that is sufficiently different from the run-of-the-mill snake medicines to merit individual consideration. This treatment involves injections of human chorionic gonadotrophin (HCG). HCG is a hormone formed in the placenta. For this reason, its presence in the urine may be used as a test for pregnancy.

HCG is fervently advocated by a number of fat specialists because it is supposed to have unique fat-mobilizing properties. Some suggestions of fat-mobilizing effects were obtained in early animal experiments with HCG. Unlike the other antifat pills, HCG cannot be taken orally. It must be administered via regular injections. An occasional shot in the bottom and your fat virtually washes down the drain. Because it requires visits to the injector on a weekly basis, it is one of the most expensive of the current crop of diet miracles. This of course does nothing to hurt its status among the antifat merchants. After all, anything that expensive and exotic sounding must be good. At the very least, it is good business.

Study after study has yielded a uniform picture of the worthlessness of HCG in bringing about weight loss. In spite of these repeated demonstrations of its ineffectiveness, HCG is as widely used as ever. Sometimes it's packaged along with other snake medicines, such as vitamins and gland extracts, but the end result is always the same. Placebo plus placebo still equals placebo. The mathematics of the addition of zeroes is simple. In the end the dieter loses. Perhaps the only redeeming feature of HCG is that it does not appear to have any of the nasty side effects some of the other ineffective agents have.

The notion that placebo plus placebo still equals placebo merits remembering. Applying this equation to any of the current crop of miraculous diet pills and potions will save you a lot of bother. It seems that, for the moment, the miracle merchants have run out of totally new ingredients. As a result they are forced into renaming combinations of all the old ones. Here is a very incomplete list of a few of the miraculous substances that are at this very moment being repackaged and renamed for launching into the ever-hungry marketplace.

- Kelp
- Seaweed
- Ascophyllum
- Vitamins

- Cider vinegar
- Tryptophan
- Lecithin
- Ginseng
- Garlic
- Royal jelly
- Amino acids

The next new diet pill that is the latest amazing discovery (or perhaps a rediscovery of an ancient secret) is certain to contain some combination of the above ingredients. They will probably be described as *bio-, natural, organic,* or *herbal.* These are new buzz prefixes that indicate to the customer that the enclosed product wears a white hat. *Chemical, artificial, synthetic,* and *alien* indicate the players on the other side. In fact, some of these individual ingredients are wonderful for all sorts of things. I particularly like garlic. However, none is any good for promoting weight loss. Compounding ineffectiveness is not going to change the overall picture no matter what the stuff is called—caveat emptor.

SILLINESS

Worthless pills and potions by no means exhaust the possibilities for diet craziness. Human inventiveness in the face of huge potential profits is formidable. Some of the diet pills discussed above had some real potential for doing what they claimed, whereas others had little or no such potential. The procedures and paraphernalia that we will discuss here have absolutely no valid principles of operation other than greed, gullibility, and ignorance.

There is a significant shift in the nature of the new products' claims to miraculousness. This new approach can be typified by a brochure for a new preparation that says it is "the key to weight loss." This brochure describes how awful it is to be fat and even presents some graphic evidence for the decline in basal metabolism with age. Lastly, it describes the product they are selling, which is simply a combination of old and familiar placebos. What is really clever about their pitch is that, apart from the leader phrase "the key to weight loss," they make absolutely no claims at all that their product will in any way facilitate weight loss!

This sort of understatement or evasion is extremely clever marketing. It neatly allows customers to fill in the blanks with their expectations of the product. More important from the producer's standpoint is the fact that they cannot be held liable for making any false claims.

Much of the crazy paraphernalia being pressed on fat people has the effrontery (and good sense) to simply present itself along with some information about fatness. They let the suckers draw their own conclusions. P. T. Barnum never realized that it would all become so easy. He lived in an era when the con artists had to go out and find their marks. They then had to carefully make their pitch in order to maximize the chances of scoring while minimizing the chances of running afoul of the constabulary. Now the marks deliver themselves, and the cons don't have to worry about the law, since it is no longer necessary for them to make any claims at all.

This category includes some of the most far-fetched ploys ever to extract money from anyone. They reillustrate the fact that the gullibility of the diet public cannot be overestimated. There appears to be a frontier line in this twilight zone beyond which increasing bizarreness enhances the appeal of the snake medicine. Elementary rules of logic are not simply to be ignored, they should be flagrantly violated. Once again fairness demands stating that often the individual sums extracted by the wild and woolly gadget merchants are rather small. However, since none of these hustlers offers even a semblance of a real weight loss effect, their products are expensive at any price.

How about an earring to lose weight? They are available in many health food stores right now. Their secret apparently lies in their tying the fat person into the cosmic pool of weight-loss energy. Judging by the worldwide increase in fatness, it appears that this cosmic pool is becoming more of a puddle. On the other hand, you don't see many fat punks. This could perhaps indicate that the earring is really on the right track, but that straight citizens are just using inadequate doses. It may be that it requires three or more earrings to be effective.

Just what the secret of the earring is eludes me. The cardboard packaging is a little short on text. The shape seems to be a simple circle, so perhaps the answer lies in the exotic metal out of which it is made. Alas, even this hypothesis doesn't work, since the price is too low for the metal to be very exotic. In addition, some of them are plastic. Who are they kidding?

It is some small amount of consolation to know that the earrings do not appear to be kidding many people at all. The cashier in my local health food bulk warehouse confides to me that they have not been a hot seller. I suggested that the problem may lie in the fact that they are on the same rack with the organic chewing gum and herbal acne cream. She agreed that the earrings probably can't stand the competition, and if the boss says it's okay, they should be moved by tomorrow.

One of the fads of the 1970s was acupuncture. You may remember that in some countries the practitioners of this ancient Chinese art ran afoul of the law—the medical professionals get upset about other people sticking pins into their customers. This gave birth to acupressure, which is essentially noninvasive acupuncture. If you practice acupressure, you are pretty much beyond the reach of the law just about anywhere.

Another attractive aspect of acupressure is that it does not require your indoctrination into the fascist, orthodox medical establishment. Of course, it is the vested interests of the orthodox medical profession that seek to repress the light of acupressure. Each new acupressure clinic means one less Mercedes in a doctor's garage. No wonder doctors are so frightened.

Acupressure does not require years and years of plugging away in some dreary medical school. Innocent people are led to believe that the only real teaching at medical school concerns how to get a big mortgage and a middle-class spouse. In contrast, acupressure is primarily learned out there in the college of hard knocks in the school of life. It is not so much a body of knowledge as it is an attitude toward life.

A little orthodox medical knowledge is not a severe drawback in the alternative medical community, but it does give the practitioner a certain amount of taint. The only way of convincingly demonstrating that one has broken the shackles of Western medicine is to take up rolling your own cigarettes. Acupressure really requires thoroughly unfettered souls who ride bicycles and sneer at Mercedeses.

Acupressure has an unfortunate history because, like all sorts of half truths that get into the hands of militant amateurs, it has been grossly oversold. It would appear that, in many branches of orthodox medicine, there is a role for techniques related to acupressure. There is some understanding as to the mechanisms of its action. It is not very magical at all.

Acupressure is also not very powerful. Medicine in China is steadily moving away from its previous heavy reliance on such techniques, simply because they are not very effective. The old Chinese medicine is not that bad, it's just not that good either. Responsible practitioners of Chinese medicine are much more modest in their claims as to what their techniques can do. The gross hyperbole occurs mainly in the Westernized variety of Chinese medicine.

There is no reliable evidence that even remotely suggests that pressing, pinning, or vibrating any part of the human body will facilitate weight loss. This absolute lack of evidence stands in startling contrast to the absurd claims of the devotees of this approach. There are clinics all over the place that promise that with a few pricks or prods your fat will disappear faster than mung beans. They, of course, are merely traveling the well-worn path of promising weight loss with no effort. Some of them throw in a philosophical overhaul for free.

Weight loss with no effort is made even more effortless by the fact that with acupressure you are not bothered by hunger pangs when you diet. Here is where we get very close to the core secrets of this pitch. Hunger is suppressed simply by applying firm pressure to your *ting kung*. The *ting kung*, as any fool knows, is the nineteenth point of the small intestine.

If pressing the *ting kung* really suppressed hunger, the starving Chinese of the not-so-distant past would be commonly depicted as pressing a small area just in front of their ears. The fact that this easily recognized posture seems to have entirely eluded painters, photographers, and other chroniclers of the passing scene for millennia leaves me a bit skeptical.

If you need any further indication of the rampant charlatanism masquerading behind this weight-loss fraud, take a look at some of their literature. Like all the hustlers in this arena, they ring in every other tired old remedy that has been shown to be ineffectual elsewhere. They have their own diets, pills, and gadgets, the only difference being the packaging in Oriental wrap.

One fairly well-publicized practitioner of the chow mein school of slenderness claims that with his program you do not lose weight. I was about to slip into some grudging admiration for his honesty when I read the next paragraph. It states that on his program you do not lose weight, you only lose fat! This miracle indicates either that fat is weightless or that the pinning process makes muscles to replace fat. If there were the slightest element of truth in this, the sports world would be revolutionized overnight. The absurdity of this nonsense is indicated by the total lack of perforated Olympians.

Diets, pins, potions, and pummeling constitute about as massive an attack on fat as is possible. Alas, the only part of the entire edifice that holds any water at all is the diet scheme he presents. Unfortunately, even his diet is no better than scores of others that are available for free and without all of the mumbo jumbo. Oriental philosophy may be the path to spiritual enlightenment, but it does not have much to offer in terms of weight loss.

All the fat-attack procedures discussed so far have shared a common element of being indirect. Diets, exercise, psychotherapy, weight-loss groups, pills, potions, and acupuncture all attempt to extirpate fat in a rather oblique manner. The very failure of these indirect slimming procedures has increased the attractiveness of procedures that take the bull (fat) by the horns and wrestle it into submission. There's no pussyfooting around here. These techniques mean business. Besides, there is always a lot of gratification to be had by hand-to-hand combat with such a long-standing adversary.

There is truly a wondrous array of techniques for directly attacking fat. They range from the old favorites of steam baths and massage to high-tech fat-dissolving creams and electrical muscle stimulators. These techniques share a number of common features besides their directness. One common feature is that they are all either low-effort or no-effort procedures. The weight-loss aspirant is acted upon by external agents and pretty much just sits there and enjoys or endures it. All they require is the will to win and a fistful of money. The financial ante is raised considerably here. A full frontal attack does not come cheap.

Ultimately, of course, financial considerations are totally unimportant for many people. They are interested in results at any price, financial or otherwise. No one has yet explicitly offered a Faustian exchange ("we take your fat and your soul together—no muss, no fuss, no bother"), but it would probably do well. In fact, Dr. Faust's eternal fat remover is too good to miss out on. Patent it quick.

What results do the direct procedures have to offer in return for their rather high prices? The answer is that apart from dividends to the merchants, the direct-fat-attack procedures have absolutely nothing to offer. They are based upon assumptions that range from the rather silly to the completely ludicrous. None of them works.

The typical French pharmacy has at least two and often three slenderizing creams or lotions prominently displayed in its front window. In fact, it is rare to see anything else in such windows anymore. The creams combine chemical heating, muscle stimulation, and fat-dissolving properties all in one expensive preparation. At these prices you would expect more than just effortless slenderizing, and you get it. They promise to remove cellulite and age wrinkles, clear the skin of blemishes, make you more supple and lithe and improve your sex life. One of them even throws in a sun tan just for good measure. Such wonders have not been extracted from a bottle since the days of Aladdin.

The cream and lotion merchants are not shy about claiming results. Their advertisements usually have a significant smattering of numbers indicating the sorts of weight loss that can be achieved with their balms. These figures are always closely juxtaposed with a full-length and sometimes full-size picture of a gorgeous woman who clearly got that way through using their product. What they neglect to provide are any real data that support their claims.

Providing solid data to back up the claims of those with commercial interests is the dreary work allotted to scientists and physicians. Alas, nobody outside of the magic-balm business has provided even the slightest shred of evidence suggesting that these products have any weight-loss effects at all. In spite of this minor niggle (they do not work), it is business as usual. I wonder how long it will be before the French pharmacies find something new for their windows? When they do, it's an odds-on bet that it will be another beauty-through-slenderness product.

The reasons why these balms do not and cannot cause weight loss is that fat is not mobilized by rubbing something on it. Actually, this is not totally true. There are some hormones, such as glucagon, that do have significant fat-mobilizing effects, but they are far too dangerous to use like this. Glucagon is wildly expensive, and even for scientific purposes it costs many thousands of dollars for a mere spoonful. Can you imagine the price if it were ever to be used by the antifat hustlers?

Further, even if the wonder balm did have a real ingredient as opposed to placebo in it, rubbing it on the skin would affect only the skin. Skin creams rarely even penetrate to the immediately subcutaneous (beneath the skin) fat, let alone to the deep major fat deposits. You don't use aspirin cream for a headache. The very most you could hope for with any of these products is thin skin!

Fat is only mobilized to be used for energy. This is essentially what glucagon does. Thus the only way that any pill, potion, or cream can work is to increase energy expenditure. At the moment there is no safe or even very effective way to do this. A number of drug companies are working actively on this problem and, from time to time, encouraging preliminary reports appear in the scientific literature.

If, for example, brown fat could be safely activated on an overtime basis, fat would certainly melt away. However, at the moment this sort of action is a long way from commercial viability. If and when this sort of product does appear, you can bet that it will not require any life-size posters of curvaceous women or silly promises to sell it. They probably won't even package it with a suntan lotion.

Once you have come to grips with the inescapable notion that fat only disappears by being used, many of the other wonder treatments become instantly absurd. Take, for example, massage. Pinching, kneading, pounding, pummeling, and generally harassing your fat deposits may make them angry, but it won't make them go away. If there were any sense in this notion, people would have skinny bottoms. Mechanical activation, irrespective of its philosophical heritage, does not cause fat to be used. Unless your fat is used today, you will still have it tomorrow.

The very same considerations apply to steam baths and body wraps. The latter is really just a space-saving steam bath at an exorbitant price. The same goes for saunas, heat lamps, and, of course, heat creams. The very most these things can do is cause a small increase in energy expenditure in order to thermoregulate in a hot environment. However, even this very small increment in energy expenditure is more than likely to be canceled out by the fact that during these treatments your physical activity is usually greatly reduced. With the body wraps there may be a small additional increase in energy expenditure caused by the fact that you look so ridiculous.

The last performer to appear in this fool's opera is the electrical muscle stimulators. These are not uniquely French, but they do seem to do particularly good business in France. The French have made them into quite an export business. One of the most remarkable things about these gadgets is their absurd prices. But, then, French luxuries wouldn't really be French without a high price tag.

The logic behind these devices is quite simple. They use bursts of fairly low-intensity electrical pulses to cause muscle activation. The essential prinicples involved in the electrical activation of muscles are among the oldest principles of physiology. The electronics and rationale involved in stimulating muscles have been thoroughly developed for noncommercial uses in research. The high cost of the commercially available gadgets is due to two main factors. One is the cost of providing a lot of extraneous knobs and flashing lights. The main cost factor is undoubtedly the astounding profit margins.

These devices promise the beneficial effects of jogging without your having to get all sweaty and uncomfortable. For this reason and because of their high cost they are primarily targeted at busy executives. Muscle stimulators can be used in the privacy of your own home or board room. Apart from their high cost they seem almost too good to be true. Unfortunately, the last statement is about the only thing about them that is true.

The increase in energy expenditure caused by passive muscle stimulation is less than that caused by picking your nose. You don't get sweaty or uncomfortable because you do not use enough energy to invoke sweating and the host of other events that let you know that you have been exercising. The muscle stimulators reillustrate one of the main principles of the contemporary weight-loss scene. You can't get something for nothing, no matter how much you pay.

As we discussed in chapter 6, genuine exercise is not a good way to lose weight. However, grunting, groaning, and panting may well have other benefits for one's health and well-being. The battery-powered executive variety of pseudo exercise offered by muscle stimulators is worthless. It doesn't help you to lose weight, nor does it have any of the ancillary benefits of real exercise. In fact, in certain cases, these gadgets may even be dangerous.

Surgery

That surgery should be the final solution to the woes of fat people is only appropriate. Surgery has been depicted as the final solution to almost every other medical condition. Many of the great advances of modern medicine have been at the prod of the surgeon's knife. Since so many problems have submitted to solution through surgery, it is not unreasonable that fatness should be among them.

Certain surgical procedures really work! Yes, some types of surgery produce massive and long-lasting weight loss. However, we will see below that even surgery is not the fat person's Eldorado. The price paid in terms of health and discomfort in order to lose a lot of weight through surgery is extraordinarily high. Unlike most weight-loss procedures, surgery can be fatal.

Perhaps the most psychologically gratifying form of antifat surgery is to cut out those ugly folds of fat. What could be more direct and to the point than to excise the blubber and throw it in the wastebasket? I imagine the knife-wielding surgeons as feeling a great sense of achievement as they hack through the helpless opposition. The background music could be "Onward Christian Soldiers" or "The Saber Dance." No one seems to have thought of having the offending mounds of fat bronzed and mounted in your front yard like a Henry Moore sculpture.

Panniculectomy, apronectomy, and all the fat-ectomy variants are woefully unsuccessful. No sooner are the patients out of the hospital than they begin their surge to regain their fat. In many cases the rate of postoperative weight gain is extraordinarily high. The high rate of weight gain indicates that these people are not just overeating. They must also be getting some metabolic help. These fat people develop the same metabolic efficiency of a person who is starving. They become unusually efficient at regaining weight. The rapid regain of the offending fat is the rule, not just the occasional exception. This suggests that fat mass is being defended both by an increase in energy intake and by a reduction in energy expenditure. It is the persistence of these homeostatic processes that is the dieter's despair.

There is one significant curiosity concerning the pattern of weight gain following surgical removal of fat. The replacement fat appears to be mainly deposited in places where the fat was left intact. For example, if you had a lot of fat removed from your belly and bottom, your new fat would tend to accumulate elsewhere. This has led to the enthusiastic suggestion that total fat removal would really solve the problem. There would be nowhere left for the new fat to go. Alas, total fat removal or even a close approximation thereof is a surgical impossibility. Fat simply occurs in too many places to be thoroughly removed.

However, there is a distinctly undesirable outcome of the tendency for new fat to grow back in the areas that were spared the surgical assault. This tendency produces some very peculiar body shapes. Imagine someone who is extremely fat, but who has a fairly normal size belly and bottom! This sort of surgery could well exacerbate any aesthetic defect that was presumably part of the reason for the surgery in the first place. It is a healthy sign of the times that fat removal is rarely used these days.

Some people who have repeatedly and conspicuously fallen off the diet wagon seek to improve their willpower by jaw wiring or splinting. These techniques are quite minor in a surgical sense and appear to attack the problem at its source—eating. Someone with his or her mouth modified in this manner can talk normally and does not appear to be obviously impaired. However, the wiring or splinting virtually eliminates the ability to chew properly. This means that the patient is pretty much limited to eating a semi-liquid diet.

Once again, the surgical substitute for willpower does not really work. Some patients learn to eat huge volumes of energy-dense liquids, such as milk shakes and ice cream. If they take this way out, it means that they lose no weight at all. In this case the operation is usually declared a failure and the muzzle is removed. Other patients do substantially reduce their food intake. This eventually results in their losing some weight. The problem occurs when the coercion is stopped (nobody stays wired or splinted forever). When the muzzle is removed, the liberated fat people rapidly eat themselves back to fatness. Oral surgical techniques for the elimination of fatness are about as ineffective as they are harmless. They can be rather uncomfortable but only rarely dangerous.

The end of the line for fat people is often stomach or intestinal surgery. These surgical procedures constitute the ultimate weapon against fat. Because of their dangers and the degree of discomfort they invariably cause, this form of surgery should only be contemplated by the truly massively obese. If you are not at least double a reasonable weight, this escape clause should never even enter the realm of possibility for you.

Unfortunately, the seductiveness of the undeniable results of gastrointestinal surgery has inevitably led to its abuse. Many dejected and repeatedly defeated dieters who are just fat, not massive, have fallen into line awaiting the surgeon's knife. This is in spite of the fact that every major medical body has sounded numerous cautions on this topic. The warnings have, to a large extent, fallen on deaf ears. Here is something that really works. In response to the increasingly strident demand for slenderness at any price, these surgical techniques are being practiced far more widely than was ever anyone's intention.

Most reputable medical centers have screening and counseling procedures that are quite effective in eliminating much of the flagrantly inappropriate use of this surgery. Their guidelines are fairly well codified and, for the most part, they appear to be strictly followed. However, as we will see below, even the most scrupulous use of rigorous selection criteria does not circumvent the basic inadequacies common to all these surgical procedures. With or without safeguards, antifat surgery does not look very good in an overall cost-benefit analysis. It is a simple question of the fat person often paying far more than the results are worth.

The fundamental inadequacy of these drastic surgical procedures is compounded by the fact that they are being increasingly done for inadequate reasons in second-rate medical establishments. One of the major findings to emerge from a number of studies of the very considerable mortality of these procedures is that it increases sharply when the surgery is not done at special centers that have extensive experience in it. Fat surgery is, in some respects, assuming the proportions of the backyard abortion business of not so long ago. The essential difference between a rusty coat hanger and a stainless-steel scalpel becomes blurred.

The technical details of the numerous gastrointestinal surgical procedures need not concern us here. Looming over all of them is the fact that they often cause massive weight loss. Huge and rapid weight loss is not invariable, but it is the usual outcome of this type of surgery. There are many cases of fat people losing 100 pounds and more! Figures like these are the pot of gold at the end of the fat person's rainbow. This is capped off by the remarkable finding that refattening after surgery is far less likely than after any other form of fat fighting.

Losing real amounts of weight by dieting is a rare phenomenon. Maintaining any significant weight loss is far rarer still. Gastrointestinal surgery appears to break all the rules by bringing about large and apparently long-lasting weight loss. Further, this modern miracle does not really require any willpower. All that is requires is the dedication and financial resources to lie down and be anesthetized.

The effectiveness of these procedures conceals a considerable amount of confusion. The logic behind the various intestinal-shortening procedures was that reducing intestinal length should result in a failure to absorb some of the energy in the diet. This would substantially reduce the tendency of any food to produce weight gains. The larger the amount of intestine that is removed, the greater the effect. Intestinal-sectioning procedures were designed to allow you to have your cake without it's ending up around your waistline. The very thought of this is dizzying to desperate dieters. However, the effects of intestinal sectioning are far more complex than a simple reduction in energy absorption.

Intestinal sectioning affects, in varying degrees, the absorption of nearly all nutrients. The very complex reductions in absorption of macronutrients and micronutrients are responsible for many of the dangerous and undesirable side effects discussed below. In fact, in many cases it appears that energy malabsorption may be only a minor factor in the overall effects of the surgery.

Further, the effects of intestinal sectioning are not restricted to producing malabsorption. It also produces a large reduction in food intake. Some of this reduction in food intake may represent a genuine reduction in hunger, but much of it is due to the long-lasting diarrhea, nausea, and vomiting that follow impaired intestinal functioning. Processes as intricate as those involved in regulating body weight are not easily defeated. Even when they are apparently subjugated, the victory often turns out to be costly. There is no such thing as a free lunch.

The aim of stomach sectioning by staples or other means is simpler. The aim here is to eliminate overeating and hunger by making the amount of functional stomach too small to hold much food. The idea is that with a small stomach you feel full faster and consequently eat less. This is not very sound logic, since is has been known for many years that normal-weight patients can often compensate for even total stomach removal by increasing meal frequency.

Healthy patients who have had a gastrectomy report feeling essentially normal sensations of hunger. As suggested above, much of the apparent lack of hunger following antifat surgery is secondary to chronic nausea. Permanent intestinal malabsorption tends to make you feel sick, and this will reduce food intake. To call this either a reduction in hunger or a genuine therapeutic effect is a serious misrepresentation of the facts.

Increased meal frequency can compensate for the reduced meal size necessitated by a smaller stomach. As a result, body weight may be regulated quite well with a small stomach or even with no stomach at all. The wisdom of attempting to reduce body weight by reducing stomach volume is akin to trying to reform a spendthrift by making him or her use a small wallet.

In spite of their theoretical and procedural differences, intestinal and stomach surgery cause weight loss by rather similar means. Either technique reduces both total food intake and the efficiency of nutrient absorption from the gastrointestinal tract. The combination of these two effects results in a marked negative energy balance.

The inevitable result of negative energy balance is weight loss. There is no way to circumvent this fundamental physiological truth. What is different here is that this is a rare case of physiological processes conspiring to facilitate weight loss. The main theme of dieting is, of course, exactly the reverse. Normally, physiological regulatory mechanisms act to inhibit weight loss. This is the main source of the dieter's despair.

The fact that the weight loss is seen as desirable at any cost illustrates just how desperate the fat community is. It is a sad truth that both of the major forms of antifat surgery tend to exact a terrible toll on nonfat body tissue. Although the aim of these procedures is to shed fat, they also tend to cause serious muscle wastage. Up to 50 percent of the short-term weight loss following gastrointestinal surgery may be muscle.

This muscle wastage reverses substantially over time, and there is usually a recovery of most of the lost muscle. There is nevertheless a lingering suspicion that this sort of prolonged assault on body muscle may cause permanent damage. It is an interesting sidelight that the stomach procedures seem to be even worse in this respect than the intestinal procedures. This is important because in several other respects, stomach procedures, particularly stapling, appear to be better tolerated than intestinal surgery. Stomach stapling is now the most widely used form of antifat surgery.

Evaluating the overall worth of the surgical procedures is much more difficult than it should be. The reasons for this difficulty are familiar. For the most part, evaluating the success of antifat surgery is done by the surgeons themselves or those working in close collaboration with them. Since these operations have such a high mortality, any surgeon who advocates this form of treatment is under very strong pressure to produce unqualified "successes." When this type of surgery is a success at all, it is invariably a highly qualified success. Unfortunately, the manifest qualifications often appear to be lost sight of in the mad scramble to lose weight.

The analogy here with psychosurgery is all too apparent. The use of neurosurgical procedures as a therapy for psychological problems has frequently been judged to be quite successful. However, the rosy view of psychosurgery is almost invariably that of the psychosurgeons. Independent observers and the patients themselves have a much more negative view. This distinctly one-sided reporting does not imply any dishonesty, it merely shows that under certain circumstances true objectivity is a very elusive goal. This general lack of objective evaluation makes the real value of these procedures difficult to estimate. It is a common characteristic that procedures that are difficult to evaluate usually do not have much to offer. If they were really as good as their proponents claim, the disinterested observer would not have to dig nearly so deep to uncover what is going on.

The following discussion of the darker side of antifat surgery almost certainly underestimates the case against these procedures. For example, many unsuccessful patients simply drop out of postoperative evaluation procedures. In other cases, a string of bad results is simply not likely to be considered as meriting publication. This self-censoring procedure would greatly reduce the probability of the data from many of the really unsuccessful programs ever reaching public ears.

Certainly, I have been impressed with the number of people who have sought me out to express their dissatisfaction and disillusionment with such surgery. Quite apart from the host of nasty side effects, in a surprising number of cases the surgery produces only trivial weight loss. Nevertheless, it would be inaccurate to say that these procedures are not generally effective in producing large and long-term weight loss. It does, however, appear that the "hit" rate of these procedures may not be as high as it is generally thought to be.

The amount of weight loss produced by the various forms of gastric surgery is not the same. The more radical and dangerous the surgery, the greater the weight loss that is likely to be produced. The stomach-stapling procedure, which has come into vogue, is popular largely because it appears to be less radical and dangerous than the other procedures, which actually cut into the stomach and/or intestines. We will see below that this is only partially true.

Irrespective of its safety, stomach stapling does not produce the massive weight losses characteristic of the other types of surgery. Significant weight losses are produced in only about 40 to 60 percent of the stapled patients. Further, when they do occur, the weight losses following stapling are much smaller than those produced by the other techniques. Not only that, but there is a much greater tendency for stapled patients to regain the lost weight in the longer term.

Even granting that the reports of the gut surgeons are perfectly unbiased and totally representative, these techniques still remain pretty frightening. Reported mortality rates vary from nil to around 15 percent. Most of the deaths occur during, or very shortly after surgery, although there are also numerous problems that may develop much later. The main causes of death read like a hypochondriac's nightmare. They include heart failure, respiratory failure, liver failure, kidney failure, pancreas failure, infections, gastrointestinal hemorrhage, and inhalation of gastric contents. These problems occur much more frequently in nonfatal forms. From 30 to 60 percent of the patients require rehospitalization within the first year!

Let us assume that the deaths represent the effects of varying combinations of bad surgery and inadequate postoperative monitoring. If that were true, the optimistic side of casting the blame in this direction would be that this pitfall could be avoided by careful choice of the right physician and hospital. This means that if you are clever (and lucky) enough, the likelihood of your dying as a result of this surgery is fairly small. All that remains, then, is the question of side effects.

The use of these surgical procedures and their side effects may be better understood when it is realized that they induce a state of chronic malnutrition. The malnutrition is the direct result of prolonged intestinal malabsorption. The effects of surgically induced malnutrition are still poorly understood. It is, however, clear that these effects are far more than minor nuisances. It should be stressed that the problems discussed below are only those that have emerged in the short term (that is, about twelve months after surgery). Since these surgical procedures are so new, there are as yet virtually no systematic data on complications that may develop over a longer period of time. This is a very large question mark.

Basically, the surgeons do not really know what they have done to these fat people. Everyone hopes that some late-developing nightmare does not develop, but at the moment, hope is all we have to go on. This seems to me to be an extraordinarily naive approach. Thousands of people have been subjected to immense short-term stress and discomfort and as-yet-incalculable long-term hazards simply to lose weight. There is a very real question here whether the cure is worse than the problem.

It is well documented that the massive weight loss following antifat surgery usually results in lowered levels of cholesterol, triglycerides, and blood pressure. It may also lower insulin levels and improve insulin sensitivity. All of these effects are clearly desirable for good health if they were at unhealthy levels in the first place. However, it is also well documented that these beneficial effects are superimposed on a background of long-term, or maybe even permanent, nutritional problems. Since many of the massively obese who are driven to surgery already have substantial health problems, this group is likely to be particularly susceptible to any nutritional inadequacies.

The essential piece of information that is conspicuously missing is whether the overall health and longevity of the massively obese is improved by the surgery. Although the above indicators are suggestive of a health improvement, they are really a trade-off against a large number of negative health factors. It is by no means clear whether this trade-off results in a net effect that is positive or negative.

Let us consider a desperately fat patient who has been operated on successfully and is still alive to experience the full impact of gastrointestinal surgery. We will also assume that she (about 75 percent are women) is losing a large and gratifying amount of weight. If she were not losing much weight, she would also likely not experience many side effects, so she would not be of much interest in this particular argument. The essential picture is that if you lose a lot of weight, you are likely to suffer a lot of side effects.

One of the first problems the patient would encounter is diarrhea. A typical result is from ten to fifteen movements a day. Besides being annoying and embarrassing, the diarrhea often causes chronic irritation and infections. This problem fortunately declines over time and may be moderated with medication. However, the diarrhea is frequently very persistent. About 25 percent of the patients still have it one year after the operation and about 15 percent still have it two years later.

The diarrhea is more than just an annoyance. Besides leading to irritation and infections, the liquid bowel movements result in a large loss of electrolytes. This loss, particularly the loss of potassium, produces all sorts of neuromuscular problems. Unless it is rapidly and effectively treated, the electrolyte loss may lead to convulsions and death. This is why dysentery is always so feared in times of warfare. Consequently, many of these patients must take regular potassium supplements and require frequent medical examinations for a long period of time. In some cases, the surgery has to be reversed in order to spare the life of the patient.

Another side effect that is partly related to the electrolyte imbalances caused by the surgery is persistent nausea and vomiting. This is undoubtedly partly responsible for the large reduction in voluntary food intake that typically follows these operations. Although good statistical data are lacking for this problem, it appears to be about as frequent and persistent as the diarrhea. Besides their obvious dangers, persistent diarrhea and vomiting also produce a severe reduction in the quality of anyone's life. If persons lose enough weight to consider resuming a normal social life, they may well be prevented from fully achieving this aim by difficulties in controlling their orifices.

In one form or another, all of these patients suffer malnutrition. This malnutrition contributes to the diarrhea, nausea, and vomiting discussed above. It also has a number of other unpleasant effects. Inadequate absorption of proteins causes hair loss as well as numerous internal effects. The protein deficiency means that any pregnancy during this period is likely to lead to mental retardation in the child. For this reason, women are strongly advised not to conceive until well after any gastrointestinal surgery.

The malnutrition is also reflected in reduced absorption of fat-soluble vitamins. This places such patients in that very small group of people who can genuinely profit from taking vitamin pills. In fact, for them it may be a real necessity. Fortunately, this problem is usually relatively transient. Vitamin absorption appears to return to fairly normal levels within a year or two postoperatively.

One of the numerous internal problems caused by surgically induced malnutrition is the formation of kidney stones. This is seen in about 10 to 20 percent of all of these patients. This problem is relatively persistent and requires that the patients adhere to a diet low in oxalates. Alas, this may mean the long-term or even permanent abstinence from a large number of tasty and healthy foods: carrots, celery, nuts, berries, and many types of greens, not to mention Coca-Cola and tea.

Perhaps the most frequent and difficult complication of gut surgery is liver disease. Within a year or two of the surgery at least 90 percent of the patients with intestinal transections develop one or more pathological conditions of the liver. The problem is less frequent with the stomach operations, but it is still very common. The basic problem appears to be fatty infiltration of the liver, but there are also a number of other structural changes that have been reported.

The usual pattern of the liver changes is that they are initially pronounced and gradually improve over time. However, there are many exceptions to this rule. Quite a few patients either do not improve or even get worse over time. Since liver failure is fatal, this is one of the main reasons for reversing gut surgery. The liver problems are particularly difficult to deal with since they may develop quickly and unpredictably. Further, the condition may be quite advanced before the patient starts really to notice it. This is only one of the reasons why any form of gut surgery requires years of frequent medical examinations. It is far from a simple matter of your coming out of the anesthetic and walking off happily into a sunset of thinness.

Although it is now clear that stomach stapling generally produces fewer problems of the sort described, this procedure carries with it its own unique difficulties. One is that the staples are quite prone to being dislodged. Besides being very painful, this of course requires a new round of surgery to fix the errant staples. It is more difficult than one might expect to keep staples fixed in moving, living tissue. The stomach is not a manila folder.

Another common problem with the stomach stapling is that it appears to cause dilation of the outlet of the stomach. This can also develop into a painful condition. However, even when it does not generate pain, the lack of a functional barrier between the stomach and the small intestine leads to all sorts of digestive difficulties. As mentioned above, these problems would be much better tolerated by the patients if they were the price to pay for losing a great deal of weight. Unfortunately, with stomach stapling this is often not the case. It produces weight losses that are much smaller and less permanent than the intestinal operations.

There is another real and frequently ignored hazard associated with all of the antifat surgical procedures. A surprisingly large number of these patients develop serious psychiatric disturbances. These disturbances are usually of a depressive nature. In some cases this may be reversed by reversing the operation, but in others the problems are more persistent. These psychiatric problems affect up to 25 percent of the patients. They are most common in males who have lost a lot of weight. It is perhaps heartening that there is a comparable number of reports of an improved psychiatric picture following gastrointestinal surgery. Clearly this sort of surgery is a major emotional event that can either ameliorate or exacerbate anyone's emotional equilibrium.

Until there are some data that are at least suggestive of an overall improvement in the health status of the grossly fat following surgery, these procedures can only be viewed as being ethically dubious at best. Is it moral or ethical to subject people to so much outright danger and long-term discomfort for what may well turn out to be only a cosmetic improvement? Even this may be an understatement, since there is the very real possibility of some long-term horror lurking in the shadows.

The most grotesque extreme to which the fear of fat has driven some people is brain surgery. We discussed some brain mechanisms involved in body-weight regulation in chapter 4. It is clear that in rats and probably many other species as well, one of the pivotal brain structures is the hypothalamus. Damage to the medial part of the hypothalamus produces overeating and obesity. In humans tumors of the medial hypothalamus produce Frölich's syndrome. The symptomatology of this very rare neurological disorder includes ravenous overeating and the rapid development of gross obesity.

Damage to the lateral hypothalamus in rats produces a syndrome that is superficially the opposite of that which follows damage to the medial hypothalamus. This sort of brain damage produces self-starvation and very rapid weight loss. In humans, this sort of brain damage almost never occurs spontaneously, since the lateral hypothalamus is actually two identical areas, one on either side of the brain. It would be a miracle if someone developed two identical tumors that destroyed only the lateral hypothalamus. If a single tumor were to invade both areas, it would be so large that the patient would be totally incapacitated anyway.

So, the first point to bear in mind here is that it is by no means certain whether the role of the lateral hypothalamus in body-weight regulation is the same in humans as it is in rats. The second point is that, even in rats, lateral hypothalamic damage produces a host of major disturbances that would be considered walloping side effects in anyone's book. These include major sensory deficits, sexual dysfunction, problems in regulating body temperature, and disturbances in sleep and heart function, to name only a few! There is hardly a major function that is left intact after lateral hypothalamic damage.

The fact that hypothalamic damage has even been tried with fat humans is scandalous. It indicates a cavalier disregard for human suffering and a formidable ignorance of basic psychobiology. Anyone who had a glimmering of what this type of brain damage does to rats would never consider trying it on humans. What is worse is that in the few cases where it has been tried, it has not even produced significant weight losses. In this respect the lateral hypothalamus of the human appears to function rather differently from that of the rat. Unlike some of the gastrointestinal surgical procedures, there is absolutely no way to repair brain damage. It is a one-way street. At the end of this street is a group of people who have had an important piece of their brains destroyed and who did not even get slim for their sacrifice.

CHAPTER 8

FREEDOM FROM FAT

There is little doubt that women are far more terrorized by the fear of fat than men are. Men are frightened, but women are paralyzed. Fat is a feminist issue. Women are under continual pressure to be slim, yet women are far fatter than men. Women start out with about 50 percent more fat than men and on top of this they are about twice as likely to become overweight. Further, women are many more times likely to develop eating disorders, such as anorexia or bulimia. These disorders come close to being exclusively feminine problems.

FAT AND FEMINISM

In chapter 1 I discussed some evolutionary reasons that appear to have loaded the dice in favor of women being fat. Women have evolved so that they are more energy efficient than men. The energy efficiency of women comes from the fact that they live in a metabolic slow lane. Women are very good at acquiring fat, and once they get fat, they are very good at hanging on to it. This has been, until very recent times, a distinct virtue. Plumpness has traditionally been a hallmark of both health and beauty.

Living in the metabolic slow lane may be partly responsible for the fact that women have always lived longer than men. Men have been forced into the metabolic fast lane by evolution.

Being in the metabolic fast lane makes men relatively inefficient in their use of energy. This is why men are relatively slim. However, the price of male slenderness may well be reduced life expectancy. Is this what women so desperately want?

Thus, it is quite clear why women are fatter than men. What is not so clear is just why women are under such incredible pressure to be thin. Why have women suddenly been saddled with a special responsibility to buck their own physiology and a million years of evolution? The brief answer is aesthetics. However, like so many brief answers, this one's brevity conceals a great deal of complexity (see chapter 1). Questions of aesthetics rarely submit to brief answers. This includes the question why aesthetics have suddenly gotten so out of synch with physiology and why this shift should so singularly affect women.

Like every other problem from nuclear war to bed-wetting, the feminist aspect of fatness has been solved by psychoanalysis. The psychoanalytic viewpoint has been plied in the international best-seller *Fat Is a Feminist Issue* (Paddington Press, New York, 1978). One of the main points of this book is that fatness is due to compulsive overeating. I have discussed this issue at length in chapters 1, 3, and 5. Briefly, there is no evidence to support this view. It is just another of the prejudicial opinions that are rife in this area. For every fat compulsive eater there is at least one slim compulsive eater. Moreover, the great majority of fat people are not overeaters, let alone compulsive overeaters. To start with such an erroneous basic assumption does not bode well for what is to follow. Unfortunately, what follows is little better. At most, the psychoanalytic explanation may apply to that small minority of fat compulsive overeaters. Considerations presented below indicate that even this limited applicability is unlikely.

There are so many flaws in the psychoanalytic approach to fatness that it is difficult to find any elements of substantial truth in it at all. The rest is so trite as to be self-evident. Study after study has shown that psychoanalysis is ineffective in treating any significant human woe. It generally turns out to be no better than talking to your hairdresser or bartender. Most of the supposedly therapeutic effect of psychoanalysis is a simple placebo effect.

Fat is a feminist issue. Unfortunately, neither the book of the same name nor psychoanalysis has done anything to illuminate the problem. Instead, the psychoanalytic approach has obscured important issues by providing pseudo answers cloaked in out-of-date, cocktail-party jargon. Worse, this approach has helped to promulgate nearly every old and wrong cliché in the fat business. Among these clichés is the fundamental issue that fat is indicative of a pathology. Fat is not necessarily a symptom of any pathology. Fat is usually just fat. What are pathological are the prevailing attitudes toward fat. These attitudes are rampant in *Fat Is a Feminist Issue*. This problem and women deserve better than that.

Eating Disorders

The antifat crusade has created major social and health problems. The antifat crusade has also done nothing to slenderize society. It has been a twofold disaster. The view that people should conform to a body-image stereotype that is inimical to their basic physiology is one of the most socially and personally destructive views of our times. The more obvious results of this crusade are epidemics of anorexia and bulimia. These serious pathologies are nearly but not exclusively confined to women.

Millions have come to loathe their own bodies and the processes of nurturing them. Food and nutrition have become the breeding ground for more forms of harmful stupidity than anyone would have believed possible. In addition to the clinical pathologies caused by the antifat hysteria, there is an ocean of unhappiness. There is hardly a single person in the developed world who has not been directly affected by this plague, which we have brought upon ourselves. What are we doing to each other?

It is impossible to discuss fat as a feminist issue without at the same time considering anorexia and bulimia. They are, in many respects, different manifestations of one problem. These disorders are both the symptoms and the instruments of the oppression of women. To find their causes does not require delving into the intricacies of the psyche. The causes are fairly clear.

If you put enough pressure on anyone for long enough, eventually he or she will cave in and develop some sort of pathology. Why certain types of pathologies emerge in some people and not in others is interesting and important, but not for the present argument. What is important for the present argument is that irrational pressure ultimately produces irrational behavior. This is the harvest we are now reaping.

Eating pathologies such as anorexia and bulimia reflect pathological attitudes toward our own bodies. These pathological attitudes probably also cause other psychopathologies that are quite unrelated to eating. At the very least, the ocean of obsessional attitudes and unhappiness caused by fatophobia must inevitably exacerbate any other physical or emotional problem. Certainly, people with the various eating disorders show an extremely high incidence of other psychopathologies. The incidence of major disturbances such as depression is extremely common, even usual, in women with eating disorders.

That fatophobia is the principal culprit in eating disorders is supported by a cross-cultural analysis. Eating disorders are much less common in societies that do not share our hysterical opposition to fat. In many countries with an abundant food supply, eating disorders are practically unknown. Further, even in the fat-loathing countries of the affluent world, eating disorders were almost unknown until very recently. All the evidence points in the same direction. We have created the problem.

Anorexia nervosa is not a trivial problem. It is far from being just a little overdose of dieting. Its appearance is distressing for two distinct reasons. One is that it is usually just the most conspicuous of a number of other emotional problems. In addition, anorexia is an extremely debilitating disorder in itself. Anorexics lead lives almost totally dominated by the pursuit of a twisted image of what they do look like and what they should look like.

It may be misleading to characterize anorexia as an eating disorder. Many anorexics are very well informed about the essentials of nutrition and health. Anorexics often appear to experience fairly normal feelings of hunger. Anorexics can eat quite normally or even to occasional excess. The problem is that they have a warped idea about what their weight should be. They can defend this weight, minuscule though it may be, by either overeating or undereating.

The anorexic behaves very much like a rat with a lesion of the lateral hypothalamus. These rats can eat normally, as indicated by the fact that they can defend their body weight against either increases or decreases. The problem with anorexics, like lesioned rats, is that they appear to defend an absurdly low, perhaps even lethally low, set-point. This is not to say that anorexia nervosa is due to a brain lesion, but it does suggest that eating is not the real pathology. Eating may simply be the mechanism for effecting a pathological change. Unfortunately, the great majority of the treatment for anorexia is largely or exclusively preoccupied with eating as the pathology.

Certainly, in the short term at least, therapy must be directed at helping anorexics to gain weight. This, of course, means getting them to eat more. It is also obvious that increased eating by itself will be of little avail unless vomiting is curtailed. However, in the long term, it would seem advisable to investigate the possibilities of trying to alter the set-point that the patients defend.

Unfortunately, establishing a new and much higher body-weight set-point for anorexics is easier said than done. In a society that so conspicuously rewards slenderness and continually reviles fatness, this is a tough pill for the anorexic to swallow. It should be, since it is the medical profession who on the one hand orchestrate the antifat hysteria while on the other tell these unfortunate few that they should be fatter.

A large part of the problem of the anorexic is a fear that if they do gain a little weight, it will lead to a complete loss of control. They have trouble discriminating the physician's advice to gain twenty or forty pounds from an injunction to blossom into grotesque obesity. Most anorexics see themselves as being incapable of stopping any upward weight spiral once it has begun. On the other hand, they often see themselves as being fully capable of staying in control of any downward changes in weight.

The very fact that they can so successfully lose weight is seen by most anorexics as a strong personal virtue. Many anorexics first reach clinical attention after competitive dieting. They join diet and exercise groups and take great pride in leading the purge parade. This is in spite of the fact that perhaps half of them are not even fat in the first place.

At one time this sort of behavior would have been considered strange or pathological. Now, however, obsessive dieting is seen almost as a virtue. Weight Watchers organized an international weight-loss competition. It sounds like the neurotic olympics. Commercial organizations and the medical profession form a united front, screeching the gospel of the fear of fat.

Anorexia is not really about eating or being fat at all. It is about the fear of fat. This fear is embedded in our language and permeates all of our social activities. It is continually reinforced by the media, commercial interests, and august medical bodies. It is little wonder that so many people are twisted and obsessed by it. In this sense only, the merchants of fear have been very successful. Until the irrational fear of fat that permeates society is stamped out, we will continue to harvest more and more human misery.

The hypocrisy of the medical profession's injunction for anorexics to gain weight, but not get fat is not simply a vacant moral attitude. It is undoubtedly responsible for much of the conspicuous lack of success of the various therapies for anorexia. It is difficult to expect anorexics to take medical advice seriously when it is based upon such conflicting expectancies. Of course they are frightened by fat—so are their doctors! It is not surprising that only about 70 percent of the anorexics who are treated are considered to be successes. Even these qualified successes often require many years of intermittent treatment and at that manage to maintain only a very low weight.

The 70 percent improvement figure for anorexics should have a familiar ring to it. It is the rate of spontaneous recovery from virtually every other psychological malady. Any treatment that does not produce results significantly better than 70 percent is operating at essentially a chance level of success. Whether the rate of spontaneous improvement of anorexics is really 70 percent is not known, but it is also not unlikely. This means that the success rate reported for various therapies of anorexia is pretty pathetic. It may well be little better than leaving them alone.

The remaining 30 percent of anorexics who do not improve due to therapy or due to spontaneous changes are not a pretty story. They are condemned to successive cycles of hospitalization and a lifelong struggle against their own obsession. Anorexia is an all-too-frequent cause of death in young women. Perhaps 5 percent of anorexics actually die of starvation. However, the real toll is undoubtedly far greater than this figure would suggest.

The continual emotional stress and malnutrition that accompany anorexia can only exacerbate any other physical or emotional problem they may suffer. Many anorexics attempt suicide. In one recent study the long-term prognosis for anorexic women was astonishingly bad. Within ten years of diagnosis, the mortality rate was more than 30 percent!

What is staggering about the 30 percent mortality figure is that it is in a group of women who were typically under twenty when their condition was first diagnosed. Only 70 percent of them lived to be thirty! Not many physical diseases are this virulent. The difference between anorexia and the more lethal forms of cancer is that for anorexia we have only ourselves to blame. We have created the problem. By continuing to adhere to absurd and antiquated views on fat and dieting, this lethal blight is being perpetuated.

Another major manifestation of our obsession with fat control is bulimia. This disorder, which literally means "ox hunger," is also sometimes called binge eating. Its main symptom is bursts of uncontrollable eating. Bulimics may eat an entire normal week's food intake in a single binge. They may literally empty a refrigerator, eating everything except the food wrappers. Often the bingers prefer "sin" food such as ice cream and cakes, but many bingers are far less discriminating.

Bulimia shares at least one central element with anorexia. They both have an overwhelming preoccupation with body weight and food. In fact, at one time bulimia and anorexia were seen as being essentially the same disorder. This is no longer thought to be the case, even though about 30 to 40 percent of anorexics also have symptoms of bulimia.

Another rather curious similarity between anorexia and bulimia is the fact that they both inhibit menstruation. With anorexia this is understandable, since menstruation requires a minimal level of body fat. With bulimics the cause of the menstrual inhibition is not clear. Most bulimics are of fairly normal weight. In a sense, the inhibition of menstruation in bulimics is adaptive. Any child conceived during prolonged laxative, diuretic, or other diet-pill abuse would be severely biochemically disadvantaged.

Bulimia is almost a pure distillate of all the myths and obsessions that surround the fear of fat. With bulimia even more so than with anorexia, the finger points directly at the fear of fat. Bulimia is apparently an entirely modern malady. It was not even diagnosed until the 1950s. However, the fact that it was a late starter does not appear to have been much of a handicap. Bulimia has really reached epidemic proportions. Not surprisingly, the epidemic is most virulent in those countries where fatophobia is most rampant.

It is significant that many people in the fat business tend to minimize the prevalence of bulimia. It is, as it should be, a source of shame to the people in the trade. This is entirely reasonable, since they are the ones who have created the environment that so richly nourishes any pathology associated with food and body weight. To staunchly defend the prevalent fatophobic environment and at the same time decry the occurrence of anorexia and bulimia is like a pyromaniac complaining about smoke. Many fat professionals do not take bulimia very seriously, because to a certain extent it is really considered just a slightly aberrant embodiment of what they see as a group of virtues.

The ambivalent attitudes on which bulimia is based are reflected in widely divergent figures on its prevalence. The most optimistic figures are that bulimia affects about 2 to 3 percent of women between the ages of fifteen and thirty-five. This is undoubtedly a very substantial underestimate, since it only includes those women who seek medical attention. It is clear that many or even most severe sufferers of bulimia never come to the direct attention of the medical profession. Even when bulimics are hospitalized, they are often diagnosed as having gynecological problems or gastrointestinal disorders.

The frequent misdiagnosis of bulimia is not helped by the fact that many bulimics are reluctant to talk about their problem. Similarly, bulimics are often very good at covering their own tracks. Jane Fonda spent over twenty years as a serious bulimic before she came out of the closet. The detection of bulimia is made even more difficult because the symptoms are not usually visible. Unlike anorexics, who are clearly given away by their emaciation, bulimics are usually normal weight. Bulimics may show large swings in weight, but their average weight is pretty much normal.

The fact that most bulimics are neither fat nor thin suggests that bulimia is a true eating disorder. This is in contrast to anorexia, which may be better characterized as a disorder of body-weight regulation. The binges of a bulimic have only a weak association with hunger. Sometimes, they are precipitated by a period of dieting, but often they occur when the patient does not feel at all hungry. Bulimics are so obsessed about inhibiting their hunger that eventually they bury it almost altogether. Eating becomes an autonomous monster freed from the normal constraints of hunger and bodily needs. The monster may be suppressed, but only temporarily. It is always there, lurking in the wings. Its entry requires only the slightest lapse in vigilance.

Over 60 percent of bulimics purge as well as binge. In their desperate fear of calories and becoming fat, they force themselves to vomit. Most bulimics further their purging by using large quantities of laxatives and diuretics. Many use diet pills and enemas as well. Bulimics represent an amalgam of every self-administered antifat remedy that is currently in vogue. During binges, many bulimics may vomit ten to twenty times a day. At first, they must force themselves to vomit by putting their fingers or a spoon down their throats. Later they often learn to vomit simply by making the appropriate muscle contractions.

The purging has a number of unpleasant consequences. One is that these behaviors greatly restrict the social life of the bulimic. It is an unfortunate sign of the times that these pathologies are becoming steadily more acceptable. It is not all that uncommon anymore to hear someone dining say, "I think I'll just make a quick trip to the bathroom to get rid of that last course." What would have at one time been considered to be a rather bizarre pathology is rapidly becoming acceptable regulatory behavior. After all, what could be more laudable than a concern with one's body weight?

Purging in all of its forms is more than just a social inconvenience. The massive food intake, along with the extreme acidity of vomit, exacts a terrible toll on the teeth of bulimics. Advanced and widespread dental decay is a frequent accompaniment of bulimia. In the extreme, bulimics can incur severe electrolyte depletion, which has occasionally led to death. The electrolyte depletion is brought about by the combined effects of vomiting, laxatives, and diuretics. This fatal extreme is rare, since most bulimics are nutritionally quite well informed. As a result, they tend to compensate for electrolyte depletion by taking potassium supplements or by eating oranges and other foods that have a high potassium content.

The increased acceptance of bulimic symptoms is clearly reflected in figures that show a much higher prevalence of bulimia than the figure of 2 to 3 percent cited above. The prevalence figures, of course, depend on how you define bulimia. Clinically significant bulimia usually refers to a recurrent and highly debilitating cycle of binging often accompanied by purging. However, just because bulimia is clinically significant is no guarantee at all that it will come to clinical attention, at least in the short term. The ultimate downstream toll of this obsessive disorder may not be apparent for years. We are still vigorously sowing the seeds of this grizzly harvest.

In addition to the clear clinical bulimics, there are many more people who are considered to be occasional or situational bulimics. In one recent study of American college students, 80 percent of the women and 50 percent of the men reported having bulimic episodes. A recent pilot study of female Australian university students suggests that 20 to 30 percent were clinically anorexic or bulimic! Figures such as these indicate that calling these disorders an epidemic is not at all an exaggeration.

Revisionist Aesthetics

It is most unfortunate that at least half of the obsessional pursuit of slenderness ultimately reduces to a single issue—aesthetics. By comparison, questions of health are almost trivial. If health were really a major element in the antifat business, most of this business would dry up overnight. The fear of fat generates far more ill health than the fat messiahs could ever hope to cure. This obsession has generated more unhealthy behavior than anyone would like to admit.

A quick scan of the numerous approaches to fighting fat reveals that, apart from radical surgery, none is effective in bringing about substantial and long-lasting weight loss. The only effective treatment, surgery, has so many dangerous and ill-understood side effects that its use is still properly regarded as both last-ditch and experimental. For the great masses of millions of weight-loss aspirants there is no effective treatment. However, if the techniques for fighting fat were simply ineffective, it would not really be so bad.

Unfortunately, virtually every one of the myriad techniques used to fight fat, with the possible exception of exercise, is either directly or indirectly harmful. The direct harm caused by dangerous diets, excessive exercise, pills and potions as well as surgery is becoming increasingly obvious (see chapters 5 through 8). These instruments of weight loss continue to exact a staggering toll in human lives and well-being.

The indirect harm caused by all of these would-be remedies is probably far greater than the direct harm they cause. It results from the fact that each antifat treatment contributes its own voice to the rising shriek of hysteria about fat. The sum of these howls is an irrational, but quite overwhelming force that is driving millions of people literally mad. Fat-related psychiatric disorders such as anorexia and bulimia are only part of the picture.

The emotional stress and stunting of pleasure produced by the fear of fat is very unhealthy. It has undoubtedly played a large role in countless episodes of psychiatric disturbances. This sort of stress must also have adverse effects on any physical ailment. Thus, the fear of fat has created a continuous assault on both our psychology and our physiology. We do not need any of this. The last thing we need is another source of anguish, particularly when it is as unjustified and unproductive as the fear of fat.

For diabetics, those with cardiovascular problems, and the massively obese, fat may well be a genuine health hazard. For this group there may be some justification in using remedies that have a certain amount of risk. It is a simple matter of balancing cost against benefits. However, quite apart from any costs, these remedies are generally ineffective. This is particularly apparent in the relatively small group of genuinely endangered fat people. Certainly, weight loss has substantial potential benefits for them. However, since the weight-loss procedures do not work, any benefits are only potential, not real. This makes for a very simple cost-benefit analysis. Attempting to lose weight has some cost and likely no benefit. You do not have to be an accountant to see that this is not a very good deal.

To make matters worse, the ineffective weight-loss procedures are advocated for millions of people who would not profit from them even if they did work. Weight loss is widely portrayed as a valid health goal for nearly everyone. The injunction to lose weight is frequently extended to those who are not the slightest bit overweight. This view is as wrong as it is destructive. Even if weight loss were a generally attainable goal (and it isn't), it is clear that it would be of benefit to only 5 or 10 percent of the population, at the very most. To advocate weight loss for the general public because of its benefits for a tiny minority makes about as much sense as suggesting that everyone take insulin because it is good for diabetics.

For many people, the obsession with slenderness ultimately becomes a question of aesthetics. This is unfortunate, since aesthetics has a particular resistance to both logic and change. It is often not clear where various aesthetic standards come from or how one goes about changing them. Until there is a substantial change in the popular view, which vilifies fat in any form and sanctifies slenderness at any cost, we will continue to be in the grip of the fear of fat. We cannot exist happily or healthily as long as we are enemies of our own bodies.

An examination of the aesthetics of fat immediately reveals a fistful of glaring anomalies. One is that men have always set the aesthetic standards for both men and women. From as far back as anyone has bothered thinking about, the beauty of women was always measured by the eye of a male beholder. This certainly reflects the fact that throughout history women have, to a large extent, been important primarily as commodities owned and operated by men. Under these circumstances, allowing women any degree of aesthetic self-determination made about as much sense as permitting horses to choose the way in which they are groomed.

There has always been more than a little similarity between the way men have treated women and the way they have treated horses. This similarity was, for a long time, quite apparent in terms of aesthetic standards. Grooming a horse has always been based around emphasizing its natural shape and textures, along with the occasional use of decorative changes to the tail and mane. Essentially the same considerations once applied to women.

Horse grooming is often complemented by decorative saddles and bridles. The styles in saddles and bridles have shown a great deal of variability over time. However, equine style in both grooming and fashion has always followed the same rule. Beauty reflects function. Consequently decoration must never compromise function. To compromise the function of a horse for the sake of decoration would be to inflict ugliness. The idea of trying to modify the shape of horses for aesthetic reasons is absurd. Any shape other than the one they come with would certainly greatly reduce their beauty, because it could only compromise their function. We have always been good to our horses.

For thousands of years, men treated women nearly as well as they did horses. This near equality has now deteriorated, and women can only aspire to the good old days. For most of the recorded human epoch, women were accorded the same degree of humanity (equinity?) as horses. Their beauty was seen as a reflection of their natural function. Their natural function was, of course, bearing children. Until perhaps the nineteenth century, a woman's beauty was synonymous with good breeding potential.

Until the nineteenth century it would have been considered absurd and ugly to compromise or even deemphasize a woman's breeding ability. It is now painfully apparent that this fundamental element of human consideration has vanished from aesthetics. It is now routinely demanded of women that, in order to be considered beautiful, they pursue insane goals of slenderness. This pursuit often compromises not only their reproductive abilities but their health and happiness as well.

The demand to be slender and beautiful is rarely made explicit. There is no need to, since it is so firmly embedded in our entire value system. Men do not need to police compliance to the absurd code they have generated. Women are far better at policing themselves than anyone else could ever be. The destructive consequences of the irrational need to conform to an impossible physical ideal are becoming increasingly apparent. We have simultaneously become the creators of an aesthetic system and its victims.

When the standards of female beauty were being codified in graphic art during the Renaissance, breeding was a serious and difficult business. Far fewer pregnancies came to term, and infant mortality was extraordinarily high. In addition, women reached menopause earlier, and both men and women had shorter lives than they do now. Reproduction was much less productive then.

So, in the beginning, beauty, sex, and reproduction were all one happy family. They were a perfectly natural alliance. Recreational sex has always been around, but an essential ingredient of the fun has usually been the possibility of children. Further, beauty was seen as an embellishment to sex, but not as a prerequisite. Many of the original sex goddesses were not very beautiful by the standards of their own or anyone else's time. Further, many of the most strikingly beautiful women portrayed in art were entirely devoid of sexual attractiveness. The Christian virgins and medieval madonnas were uniformly ethereal and asexual beauties.

With the advent of the modern age, around the end of the eighteenth century, reproduction gradually became a much less important part of sex. For the first time in history, contraception became fairly respectable. This led to the development of a new concept of beauty, in which reproductive potential had much less importance. Beauty had traditionally played a rather minor role in sex and reproduction. It now quickly expanded in importance to fill the gap left by the departure of reproduction.

It was not long before the new "unnatural" beauty (that is, not related to reproduction) formed an unholy alliance with sex. Beauty became almost the exclusive passport to sex. For the first time, beauty and sexuality became almost totally interdependent. This combination has been haunting us ever since. Until beauty is redefined in much broader terms or is no longer seen as such an imperative for sex, we will continue to be tormented. It is high time we gave ourselves a break.

No single factor has ever been as good a visual indicator of the potential of a woman to provide heirs as the presence of fat. The reproductive functions of women have evolved to tie them very closely to the presence of body fat. Menstruation in young girls does not start until a critical level of fat stores has been reached. One of the major clinical signs of both anorexia and bulimia is a cessation of menstruation. The association between body fat and reproductive processes is not an evolutionary accident.

A critical mass of fat and intact mechanisms for defending it have, until very recently, been absolutely essential for ensuring the survival of children. A mother without this capacity would be bringing an infant into a world in which it would have to fend for itself. Infants are very bad at fending for themselves. Now, the need for a robust mother is not so great, but for a million years or so this harsh reality shaped female reproductive processes.

The same realities that shaped female reproductive processes also shaped the female body. Women are designed to have much more fat than men. The complex mechanisms that have evolved to defend fat do a marvelous job. Now, in what is little more than an eyeblink of the human epoch, this exquisite machinery has been declared persona non grata and asked to leave. Dictates of beauty indicate that the old physiology is no longer welcome.

Contemporary standards of beauty are totally at odds with the way most of us (women in particular) are built. A tiny minority of the population actually meets these ideals with no particular effort. It is as difficult for most of them to gain weight as it is for most of the rest of us to lose weight. Unfortunately, the odd cases of easy, natural slenderness are depicted as the norm to which the remaining 99 percent of us freaks should aspire. For the vast majority of those who are fashionably fat, achieving even an approximation of fashionable slenderness requires the adoption of a permanent regimen of Spartan austerity.

A few people can slenderize and stay that way. That this is occasionally possible is indicated by the ranks of emaciated high-fashion models and proprietors of weight-loss salons. However, substantial and permanent weight loss is not generally possible. This is indicated by the fact that at least 95 percent of the dieting public fails miserably. There is an enormous toll exacted by the fruitless and relentless pursuit of slender beauty.

Many of the successful sylphs have gained their ectoplasmic proportions at the cost of acquiring anorexia and/or bulimia. The price paid by the less successful dieters may be less obvious, but every bit as high. Foot binding of women in the Orient vanished some time ago. Torture for the sake of aesthetics has recently been resurrected in a far more widespread and virulent form, as dieting.

Cultural transitions from one ideal body to the next have always been aided by the arts. Painting, sculpture, and, more recently, photographic media have acted to disseminate the image of what is beautiful. It is very likely that the perniciousness of the contemporary stereotypes is due to the fact that they are far more accessible than images have ever been before. For millennia, painting and sculpture were only ever seen by a minuscule proportion of the population. However, this has all been radically changed. The traditional arts are no longer of major importance for conveying aesthetic ideals. The advent of nearly universal visual media, such as magazines, movies, and television, has changed all the rules.

In the past, limited access to the graphic arts acted to buffer the effects of the stereotypes they portrayed. It is probable that for most of human history only a small proportion of the population ever knew what the ideal form of beauty was. How can you become obsessed with pursuing a standard that for you does not even exist? This is no longer the case.

The explosive increase in the accessibility of visual media means that many stereotypes are now approaching global proportions. This is particularly unfortunate, since extensive international communications could have the opposite and much more salutary effect. They could have led to a diversification of aesthetic standards. Alas, Hollywood seems to have won the day, and even much of the non-American media has humbled itself by a slavish imitation of middle-American style and values. There is hardly a corner of the globe that has escaped pan-Californianism.

Of course there have always been quite distinct aesthetic ideals for men and for women. The main difference is that the standards for men have been far less changeable and pernicious than those for women. The Greek image of a muscular Adonis is still pretty much the popular ideal of a beautiful, sexy man. The only significant changes to this venerable stereotype have been in periodic changes in hairstyles and a progressive lengthening of the penis.

The heroic males whose beauty has been perpetuated in marble are not very well hung. Beautiful, nude men are rarely venerated in stone anymore. Instead, they are photographed shimmering in body oil or trying to look petulant. But it is clear that men of nonstallionesque penile proportions need not apply. These male stereotypes are less harmful than the female stereotypes in that they are clearly not interpreted as portraying a standard to which every man should conform. They are ideals, not absolute standards. They differ importantly from female standards in the lower level of compliance they demand.

Nevertheless, men do suffer somewhat from body-image stereotyping, too. The pendulous penises of the erotic ideal males cannot be obtained by dieting or surgery. You either have one or you don't. Since most men manifestly do not have such leviathan penises, the image serves only to intensify the feelings of sexual inadequacy shared by most men. The giant penises of the contemporary sex gods simply serve to exacerbate male performance anxiety. However, the terrorism exerted by the male sex stereotype is relatively benign.

The general sexual and aesthetic diminution of real men suggested by the comparisons with the huge penises of ideal men primarily affects men. Women are much less concerned about penis size than men are. If anyone were to come up with a treatment that would guarantee monumental penis enlargement (it would probably consist of carrots, cucumbers, and zebra hormones and be called Apocalypse Now), it would be a sellout. It's been said before that women do not suffer from penis envy, men do. At any rate, men don't really get twisted very much out of shape by the lack of length or in pursuit of greater length. On the other hand, many millions of women are seriously disturbed by their obsessive fear of fat and the pursuit of slenderness.

The relative constancy of the image of the ideal male stands in marked contrast to the rapid fluctuations in the image of the ideal woman. There have certainly been some long-term trends, but superimposed on these is a bewildering array of short-term fluctuations. The rapid fluctuations in standards of female beauty are a very modern development. For example, the women of classic art were portrayed to emphasize their breeding potential. Botticelli's *Birth of Venus* shows a woman with a plump belly, as well as rather large legs, thighs, and hips. This ideal endured for hundreds of years. However, by contemporary standards, Venus simply appears to be fat.

An important difference between the standards of beauty in

classic and contemporary art concerns their relative heterogeneity. The ideal portrayed by Botticelli's Venus was perhaps typical of the times. Nevertheless, in the same period other artists portrayed beautiful women who had quite different proportions from those of Venus. Even Venus herself has been represented in many different configurations.

Reubens painted one of the fattest Venuses. Today, any woman of Reubenesque proportions is likely to be involved in every weight-loss scheme around. On the other hand, in the sixteenth century, Lucas Cranach painted a Venus who is slender even by contemporary standards. Not to fall into a rut, Cranach also painted another Venus of near-Reubenesque proportions. Beauty was idealized in classic art, but it was idealized in many different forms. This sort of aesthetic heterogeneity died some time ago. Modern standards of beauty are probably narrower and are certainly more restricting than they have ever been before. As standards of beauty became more rigid and narrow, they also took on the nastiness that is now their most striking characteristic. Aesthetics have become a universal tyranny.

A bottom-heavy, rather flat-chested woman such as Venus would be quite unattractive by the standards of today. At one time she epitomized all that was beautiful about women. Her girth and low center of gravity were all fine indicators that this woman would bear many healthy children. Her being somewhat flat-chested by modern standards would have gone unnoticed. Her breasts were large enough to suckle, besides which there were always plenty of wet-nurses to assist with feeding.

The essential features of the classic ideal of a beautiful woman began to change around the eighteenth century. At this time some distinctly odd clothing styles were developed. They amounted to a form of bondage, which permitted some minimal amount of movement on the part of the victim. Women were trussed, belted, laced, and stayed. When you start tightening all this gear, it is obvious that the displaced mass has to go somewhere. The use of mechanical coercion to produce a wasplike waist has an inevitable consequence. The displaced fat is driven upward and downward. Clothes mechanics thus discovered tits and bums. This discovery provided the major elements of the contemporary ideal woman.

Ebullient breasts and an abundance of bottom ushered in the era of the modern beauty. These signs of conspicuous opulence cost early-modern women relatively little in terms of loss of freedom or comfort. The pinched waist sometimes made them a little short of breath. If the women bent over too far, their low necklines made it likely that there would be a problem of breast fallout. Similarly, sitting down was sometimes difficult in confined spaces because of the presence of a bustle to enhance their splendor. These were relatively minor and definitely superficial inconveniences. In terms of their conduct, they were relatively unfettered by their decorations. They could eat, drink, and do fairly much whatever they wanted. Foundation garments took care of the rest. It would perhaps be more correct to say that their limitations were not imposed by aesthetics. In this sense early-modern women had a degree of personal freedom that late-modern women have abandoned.

In terms of a modification of body shape, the advent of the modern woman was a major event. The pearlike shape that had persisted for a thousand years or more was replaced by the hourglass figure. However, the popularity of the hourglass figure was relatively short-lived. The first lasting modification to the hourglass was the elimination of the bottom. The "flapper" of the twenties embodied a temporary constriction of both ends of the hourglass.

In the 1920s, female beauty was an emulation of boyish slenderness coupled with an air of abandonment and freedom. This was maybe the first time ever that a woman's freedom was viewed as anything other than a threat to males. Now the freedom itself was an integral part of her attractiveness. The flapper signified a radical departure from the past, in terms of both aesthetics and behavior. One observer remarked that the flapper image did far more than simply abandon the traditional association between beauty and reproductive potential. The flapper was positively contemptuous of the idea of reproduction. The old ways were dead. Who knew what would happen?

The flapper era was little more than a temporary recession in the rising tide of breasts as symbols of female beauty and sexuality. However, the flapper did pretty much put to rest the rise of the bounteous bottom. The great blossoming behinds of the nineteenth century did not survive the roaring twenties.

As we will see below, bottoms are only half dead.

Bottoms were not really killed off entirely by the flappers. Physiology is just not beaten that easily. However, they did introduce the first coherent and widely accepted image of a very slender woman. This image continues to torment us. Of course, in the 1920s, there was no fundamental change in female physiology or body shape. There was, however, an important change in aesthetic ideals. By emphasizing angularity and minimizing the importance of the two traditional focal points of female pulchritude, they created the image of the first really synthetic woman. This woman was synthetic in the sense that she was an explicit denial of the natural. She broke all ties with the past and was, therefore, a pure creation of the twenties. Synthetic people do not work well. We should have learned that from Frankenstein.

The popular image of the scrawny flapper was positively leaped upon by the fashion industry after World War II. Here, at last, was an ideal vehicle for the designer's clothes. The thinner the model, the less annoying flesh there was to disrupt the pure lines of his (they were almost exclusively male) creations. These times gave rise to that singularly unwholesome expression for a high-fashion model as a "clothes hanger." This demeaning term is still considered an aesthetic ideal in some circles.

Designers' imaginations led to increasingly absurd standards of slenderness. The aesthetic hyperbole of high fashion rapidly filtered down into the mass marketplace. In the 1960s, popular and comfortable everyday garments such as jeans soon became a thoroughly inhospitable environment. Style demanded Ethiopian proportions in order to look right in them. It soon became apparent that designers' fantasy lives could not be accommodated even by the almost shadowless high-fashion models, let alone mere mortals. This led to a still-very-popular tendency to portray fashions in drawings. The strokes of pens, pencils, and paintbrushes are not fettered by mundane considerations, such as having to accommodate a real human being.

While this body squeeze was taking place, breasts were going their own independent way. The desirability and form of mammary display waxes and wanes almost yearly. Breasts continue to be ignored by high fashion as annoyances, but popular fashion has its own life in this respect. Not the least reason for this is the fact that the bra business is very big business indeed.

So, while a general and radical slenderizing is taking place (this slenderizing is only in desire, the population is becoming steadily fatter), breasts pop up and down with the regularity of seasonal flowers. The message is "Lose weight but spare your knockers. You can strap them in for now, but next year they may be in fashion again." Women cannot possibly be all things, particularly at the same time. Why don't we leave women alone for a while so that both men and women can find out what they are really like?

The popular attitude toward women's bodies has now reached a new level of schizophrenic absurdity. For quite a long time now women have been demeaning themselves in the frantic pursuit of the latest whims of male aesthetic demands as orchestrated by the fashion industry. Just when women were getting used to this frenetic activity, we changed the rules again. Now no woman can possibly comply with them.

Not content with demanding of women that they pursue a generally unattainable body shape, we now demand that they pursue two at once. The fact that these two shapes are mutually exclusive is too much for anyone. Women must now have two bodies. One is for wearing clothes. This dressed body is thin, thin, thin. On the other hand, thin is still beautiful, but it is no longer sexy. Women now need a different nude body for sex appeal.

The nude woman that men want is presented in the girly magazines and cinema. Here we see sweeping curves and an abundance of breast perched ever higher and at more bizarre angles. The bottom reappears (remember I said that it was only half dead), substantial and suntanned. The contemporary sex goddess is not a reincarnation of the hourglass shape, she has a bottom, but on the hourglass scale of the nineteenth century it is rather tiny. Frank Zappa succinctly characterized the new sex goddess as having "titanic tits and sandblasted zits." Apart from the flawless complexion, the rest of this equipment just does not fit under the clothes we want our ideal woman to wear.

The problem is that two, divergent courses might be simultaneously adopted by women to be "ideal." Men want them to have one body for clothes and another for fun (men's fun, not theirs). Until someone comes up with inflatable breasts that can be instantly adjusted to suit the situation, the dual-bodies image will remain unattainable. Meanwhile of course, many more emotional scars will be created.

One reason that these suntanned female hyperboles have captured the popular imagination is the lack of clear alternatives. Most men have never seen a real naked woman until their first sexual encounter. They may have caught glimpses of their mothers or sisters in the nude, but few have ever been able to examine these stolen glimpses closely. By the time they get the opportunity for some firsthand experience with someone else's flesh, the aesthetic die may have been cast.

At this formative time, most male teenagers spend a lot of time imprinting on skin magazines. Although this likely causes no permanent deterioration of vision, it certainly does have long-term aesthetic effects. No wonder the bizarre confections popularized in paper and in films have become the fire for the popular libido. The permanence of this artificial aesthetic system is also helped by the fact that so many males spend the rest of their lives trying to hang on to that first flush of puberty.

Very few men have ever really seen a fat woman in the nude. If they have, it is likely in a comical context. Fat women are no longer supposed to be either beautiful or sexy. They are portrayed as the very antithesis of beauty and sexuality. This deficiency is not remedied much by public nudity. Fat women, in particular, do not usually bare themselves at public beaches. Their judgment of their own ugliness is usually every bit as harsh as that of the teenage skin-magazine addict. Well-established aesthetic standards generate their own policing.

Most men, particularly in the critical years around puberty, have very little exposure to female nude reality, as opposed to nude fantasy. Not only are they ignorant about what fat women look like, but they rarely know anything about ordinary, average-weight women. They have grown so used to seeing women portrayed as appendages to enormous breasts that normal women seem strange. Of course, the reverse should be true.

The unreal nature of the male image of a nude female beauty is compounded by the fact that the contemporary sex queens all share exactly the same suntan and not one of them has ever had a zit. Further, every aesthetically offending hair has been relentlessly purged from all of their nooks and crannies. Yes, even the crannies are often plucked like eyebrows in the pursuit of perfection. Real women do not look like this. Portraying these stereotypes as ideals to which all women should aspire does a great disservice to both men and women.

Fantasy has an important place in all of our lives. However, when fantasy begins to crowd out reality, we are in trouble. This is what has happened to standards of beauty and sexuality. Women who are beautiful, sexy, slender, and curvaceous have gone from being the stuff of pure fantasy to being everyday expectancies. Of course, such absurd expectancies are not fulfilled. The net result is disappointment and disillusionment for both sexes. We are badly in need of alternative aesthetic models that are less fantastic and pernicious.

Beauty and sexuality come in many more forms than our current values recognize. Unfortunately, these other forms have no place in our narrow and constricted aesthetic spectrum. The mass media and fashion industry have no room in their definition of beauty and sexuality for real people. When real people are used in the media, it is usually because the promoters cannot afford to hire fantasies. In this context, reality has developed an unfortunate association with sleaziness. Until real people who are fat, thin, and regular size come to be considered the accepted norm, we will continue to suffer the moral-aesthetic tyranny fostered by the fear of fat. We are all the poorer for it.

There is now emerging the first glimmer of what may be a new dawn. Some long-silent voices are being raised and they are saying no. A significant and increasingly vocal minority is attacking the established views on fat as a major form of oppression, particularly affecting women. Fat liberation is gaining a modicum of respect in the more mainstream strata of society. More is being heard of and from groups such as the Fat Underground, the National Association of Fat Americans, and the Fat Sisters Organization.

There have been successful prosecutions on the grounds of antifat discrimination in a number of Western countries. A few books have recently appeared that deal with the issue of being beautiful without being thin. One of the more heartening signs of change is that recently one of the sex goddesses of rock and roll (Madonna) bared all for a men's magazine. What was remarkable was not her nudity but the fact that she had no suntan and had a small but distinct roll of waist fat. She also had less than perfect skin and displayed a luxuriant growth of hair under her arms! Not only that, but she lacked the almost compulsory vacant gaze found in magazine nudes. In short, she looked suspiciously like a real woman.

These are still, unfortunately, rather isolated indications of dissatisfaction with the aesthetic status quo. They are not yet a groundswell of public opinion. In Washington, D.C., a group of feminists has formed a special support group for fat women. This group, which is called the Fat Sisters Organization (FATSO), has only four members!

Revisionist Nutrition

The general public is dreadfully worried about what they eat. It's not that eating habits are changing all that much, but worrying habits are. The fact that it is food that makes you fat is only one element in an immense paranoid structure. Even if you don't get fat, you can eat too much or too little of certain foods. This form of inadequate nutrition has been linked with the precipitation of nearly every woe that is known to or is suspected of afflicting our species. Conversely, it is widely believed that adopting the correct diet is the remedy for most or of all of these woes.

These beliefs have spawned a "new nutrition" that is a strong rejection of both traditional nutrition and traditional medicine. The basic tenet of this movement is that you are what you eat. Medicine and nutrition become one. The scope of this rejection is greater than many people imagine. It is summed up in a brief dialogue in the 1954 movie *The Wild One*. The ingenue asks, "What are you rebelling against, Johnny?" Marlon Brando replies, "Whaddya got?" This is the credo of the new health religion. Any view of the medical-nutritional establishment is bad. Any view that is alternative, natural, holistic, organic, or Eastern is good. The ineffable truths of health are in our gardens and fields now. The oracles of this people's health movement are the health food stores.

The idea of improper nutrition as the source of all our woes has been fostered considerably by antifat paranoia. Antifatism, however, only stresses the supposedly lethal effects of overnutrition. The real credit for the panic in our kitchens must go to the health food industry. They have created an unprecedented fear of what is on the end of our forks. They have cashed in handsomely on the fear that they have sown. Their profits would make an oil sheik blush. This enormous industry is built on a mass perception that we are eating not just badly but dangerously. In response to their creation and relentless cultivation of this fear they have come up with a comprehensive range of products to remedy what, they say, are glaring deficiencies.

Like many of the weight-loss entrepreneurs, the health food barons see themselves as doing well by doing good. It should come as no surprise that many of the major health food suppliers are also major suppliers of the other stuff as well. Walking on both sides of the fence is common in the fat business too. If it sells, we'll sell it. This high moral stance taken by many in the health food trade is more than a little hypocritical. It turns out that the great majority is far more interested in the healthiness of their bank balance than in the health of their customers. Business is, as always, business.

A visit to any health food store reveals uncharted new horizons for nutritional harm and healing. The merchants of mung beans can point at any illness, quickly prescribe a remedy, and proscribe various dietary agents that cause or exacerbate your woe. Not satisfied with merely eradicating all current diseases and unhappiness, they have resurrected old and sometimes nonexistent disorders. They have resurrected even more old folk remedies. Nineteenth-century almanacs are now doing a very brisk business. Should you come down with dropsy or lentigo, you now know where to go.

The book section of any health food shop contains a staggering array of nutritional quackery. It is apparent that the only criterion for offering anything for sale is whether people will buy it. Present any nonense with the appropriate incantation of *natural, holistic, organic,* and so forth, and it will be swallowed faster than alfalfa pills. Their criticism of health and nutrition establishments is often well justified. Unfortunately, their criticism is often completely unilateral. It obviously does not extend to the alternatives that they themselves offer. Most of their books and remedies defy even the broadest and most charitable definition of logic. The "Marxist-lentilists" are more at the mercy of buzzwords and hype than is the most linguistically debauched advertising executive.

There is no idea or remedy that is too stupid for the new

nutritionists. The only thing that will cause a product to be removed from the shelves of health food stores is slow sales. Their ideology strongly rejects the commercialism of the establishment. At the same time, many are more crassly commercial and amoral than the worst of the establishment villains they rail against. They have taken the classic right-wing battle cry "freedom of choice" to absurd and dangerous extremes.

Ultimately, as with any remedy, what is important about health food remedies is not their logic or lack thereof, but whether they work. Proponents of the health food cause point to herbal remedies that were in use long before there was any good reason for them to work. One notable thing about these genuinely effective remedies is that they have all been incorporated into mainstream medicine. When asked to provide evidence that any of their new prescriptions work, they are usually nonplussed and point to an example of someone for whom it was just the ticket. Usually this is someone known, secondhand, by someone else or someone they read about in the *Nuts and Raisins Weekly* or in the literature provided by the supplier of the product in question.

When the skeptical inquirer points out that second- or third-hand anecdotes or advertising claims are not a very sound basis for making a health investment, the merchant's shell really begins to close. By demanding proof, you have declared yourself to be a nonbeliever. This is anathema, since a critical element in all these remedies is faith. Of course the remedy might not work in a cold-blooded clinical trial, since the vibrations are all wrong. As for statistics, that sort of mathematical fascism is severely disruptive to good karma. You must have faith.

Why one should have faith in the health-food merchants as purveyors of health defies comprehension. Health shop employees freely make diagnoses of and dispense for countless ailments. They typically ply their trade without the impediment of any knowledge even remotely related to health or nutrition. They are often uneducated or untrained in anything else as well. The only credentials required for working in a health food shop are wanting a low-paid job and having a wan complexion and almost inaudible voice. In lieu of these credentials, elderly, caring women are quite acceptable. Usually the employees' only source of knowledge is the brochures of the very stuff they are trying to sell.

It is more than a little strange that the health-food movement, which sees itself as a reaction against authoritarian nutritional and medical orthodoxy, has become far more authoritarian than its mainstream relatives. The great majority of establishment nutritional and medical wisdom is capable of being refuted. There is always some evidence that, if it existed, would result in the demise of any of the great truths of the establishment sciences. This is not the case with health food faddism.

The alternative health gospel is just that—gospel. It is rarely open to serious questioning, and there is rarely any evidence that would shake the belief of the faithful. It is pure and simple authoritarianism. It seeks to avoid the authoritarian label and annoying issues of being right or wrong by allowing a plurality of remedies. The fact that they issue so many, often contradictory pronouncements and that they come from someone wearing denim and who speaks softly does not diminish their authoritarian nature. Nor is quantity of remedies any substitute for quality. When any idea seeks to isolate itself from questioning and evaluation, you had better put your caveat emptor on full alert.

The perfect example of this is the bogus cancer cure laetrile. Laetrile is one of the brand names given to an extract of apricot kernels. According to its devotees, the main active ingredient of laetrile is cyanide, which, according to their logic, is what kills cancer cells. This treatment has all of the cachet of being a "natural" product and having a simple, understandable mode of action. It has made people millionaires.

The only thing that laetrile lacks is effectiveness in combating cancer. This should not be much of a surprise, since the logic on which it is based is not only terribly simple, it is just plain terrible. Certainly, cyanide and a great many other substances have an anticancer action when given in high enough doses to cell cultures in test tubes. That, of course, is not enough.

The downfall of the minimal logic in laetrile is that humans are not simple cell cultures, nor are they enclosed in glass. Cyanice doses even approaching those that are effective in test tubes are extremely lethal in humans. Large enough doses of laetrile could well kill cancers by the shortest route of all, by killing the patient. You could achieve this same end by massive doses of laxatives, but nobody seriously suggests this as a cancer cure. Actually, the last statement is not strictly true. Fervent advocates of detoxification through enemas see their pastime as central in the cure of many diseases, including cancer. Laxatives are the next best thing to a large rubber syringe full of warm water, but syringes are a whole lot more fun.

The appealingly simple logic of poisoning cancer with natural toxins has repeatedly been shown to be a dead end. Alas, in many cases of cancer this is a literal truth. In Ireland one of the time-honored folk remedies for cancer is the local application of a bitumen paste. This same paste is used with some effectiveness in combating household pests. The anticancer tar has no therapeutic effect at all, but it is very toxic. The disfigured victims of this cruel quackery may still be seen, particularly in rural districts. Many more mutilated corpses who succumbed to the joint effects of their cancers and the tar are buried evidence.

In spite of numerous studies showing that laetrile has no more anticancer effect than any other placebo, the demand for it remains strong. It remains strong because its importers will not accept any data that their nostrum is ineffective. Consequently, they will not let such negative propaganda reach the ears of their acolytes. It is to their additional discredit that these charlatans present themselves to their followers as the only source of truth. Moreover, they maintain that it is a matter of a fundamental liberty to choose any treatment, even if it is ineffective. This is like extending the freedom of speech to include shouting "Fire" in a crowded theater.

Each one of the cancer sufferers who is duped by laetrile and its companions necessarily does not receive some other legitimate treatment that at least has a hope of working. This is always the danger with any pseudo-medicine. Antilaetrile legislation proved quite ineffective in stemming the spread of laetrile "therapy." The main effect of the legislation was to drive laetrile underground and boost the price. Mexican cancer clinics, which are parodies, are packed with desperate and dying laetrile takers.

There is not a single shred of evidence that is even remotely suggestive that laetrile is a genuine therapeutic agent in any species, at any dose. Nevertheless, many American states have recently passed prolaetrile legislation. To restrict choice in any manner smacks of big brother and totalitarianism. Not surprisingly, many of the key figures in the American laetrile movement are members of ultra-right-wing political groups, such as the John Birch Society. I wonder if they have considered the chilling possibility that laetrile, like fluoridation, is a communist plot to corrupt the precious bodily fluids of the American nation. If this is the case, the international communist conspiracy has succeeded in putting its most ceaseless enemies in its own pocket. Gentlemen, pause and think for a moment.

Prodded by a slowly growing public awareness that laetrile is not much good for anything, other enterprising charlatans have adopted quack ploy number 2. That is, if your product is not selling well (forget whether it works or not, because none of them do), you must make it more distinctive in the crowded marketplace. One time-honored way of doing this is to combine it with others that have a certain amount of pull on their own. Here again, value can only be measured commercially. The term *valuable commodity* really means anything that has not been a failure long enough and conspicuously enough to have developed a public image of being a "loser."

Laetrile has been commercially reinvigorated as part of a package that calls itself total metabolic therapy. This new wonder is a cocktail of nearly every transient hope that ever beguiled a sick person. Its ingredients are a litany of homilies (detoxification, rest, and a positive mental attitude) and vitamins of both the genuine and the dubious variety. There is something for everyone, with the notable exception of the patient. This farrago of nonsense is completed by the fact that it can only be practiced by believers! The last point is the catch-22 as far as validating this snake medicine. Since anyone who would seek to evaluate this regimen objectively is, by definition, not a true believer, anything he or she comes up with is not to be trusted.

When threatened with prosecution on the grounds that laetrile is a drug and as such should be regulated by the medical profession, some of the laetrile fraternity took a new and slippery tack. They disavowed any claims that laetrile is a drug. They made it into a vitamin! Laetrile is not the first, nor will it be the last, health hustle to ride on the vitamin train. Probably no single element has contributed so much to the deterioration of nutritional rationality as the vitamin. Vitamins were first recognized as a nutritional entity and named in 1911 by a Polish biochemist with a name that would have delighted W. C. Fields. The father of vitamins was named Casimir Funk.

Until the discovery of vitamins, nutrition was a very simple business. Even a child knew the rules, since they were just common sense. If it looks good, tastes good, and makes you feel good, it is healthy and nutritious. Vitamins changed one important aspect of this view, and as we will see below, the sciences of epidemiology and toxicology changed the other.

The discovery of vitamins suggested that foods that were apparently good could be seriously lacking in vitamins. Their vitamin deficiency made them fundamentally nonnutritious. Then toxicologists challenged the assumption that if something made you feel good, it must be good. They showed us that what we thought to be healthy food may make you feel good in the short term, but in the long term it may lead to all sorts of ill health. Nutrition was far more than just common sense.

What was disturbing about these discoveries was that the new dimensions in food were not detectable by odor, sight, taste, or touch. This meant that you could no longer trust your own good sense in choosing food. Not only that, but since there were no agreed-upon standards as to how much of any of the vitamins were required for good nutrition, you didn't even know how much to supplement your diet with. The only safe way out was to take lots of them.

The fear of undetectable and malevolent forces in what we eat was given additional, if indirect, motivational force by the international crusade against smoking. For centuries smoking was thought to be good, clean fun. Suddenly, it appeared that after all of these hundreds of years, every medical person worth his or her salt was loudly decrying the hazards of smoking. Smoking has been strongly associated with nearly every health horror that lurks under any hypochondriac's bed. Moreover, this was no passing scare, as was the case with artificial sweeteners.

Year after year the evidence accumulated. By anyone's data, smoking either caused, precipitated, or exacerbated almost every human malady. The number of dissenting voices steadily diminished to where now there are few people, even in the tobacco industry, who will argue strongly against the antismoking data.

The most common tack taken by these people is that smoking has become a matter of freedom of choice.

Millions of people gave up smoking. It was clearly an obvious way of reducing the risk of cancer and other diseases as well. The only group that currently smokes more than ever is young women, most of whom see it as a way to keep their weight down. For the present argument, the important aspect of the whole smoking issue was that it finally and unequivocally showed that something that felt good might be really unhealthy.

Now, just as you begin to think you have yourself covered by quitting smoking and taking lots of vitamins, someone discovers a new vitamin that is more essential for good health or more destructive to disease than the last. Vitamins breed faster than rabbits. With our health at the mercy of so many unseen and malevolent forces, it is little wonder that food paranoia is rampant. A majority of the Western world believes that no matter how healthy one's diet is, it should be supplemented by vitamins.

At least 99 percent of the lore about vitamins is sheer hokum. There is no evidence that anyone who is reasonably healthy and who eats even a fairly balanced diet needs vitamin supplements. For diseases and for people who eat glaringly unbalanced diets, vitamins may be desirable or even necessary. The people who could really profit from them probably constitutes only a small percentage of the population of most Western countries.

This means that at least 50 percent of the population of the overdeveloped world is being conned. That adds up to hundreds of millions of suckers. They are being stampeded by a mass miseducation program into regularly taking vitamins that cannot possibly help them. The reasons that vitamins cannot help them is that these people have no vitamin deficiency to correct. There is a striking parallel here with injunctions to lose weight. The majority of the population is regularly told that they would be healthier if they lost weight. In fact, weight loss would only benefit about 10 percent of the population. As with any treatment, just because it is good medicine for some people does not mean that it is good for everyone. Logical niceties such as this tend to get lost in the current nutritional hysteria.

Whereas very high doses of some vitamins such as A and D

are dangerous, most excess vitamin intake is simply excreted. The affluent nations have very expensive urine. It became still more expensive during the vogue of "megavitamin" therapy. This is yet another application of the logic that if a little is good and more is better, then buckets must be wonderful. Linus Pauling, of Nobel Prize fame, reckoned that if you gobbled up enough vitamin C, you could cure the common cold. Further, if you regularly colored your urine in this manner, you might even be able to avoid colds altogether.

As a result of his fervent belief and the immediate capitulation of most of the rest of the world (few dissenting voices were heard), vitamin C sales skyrocketed. The slightest sniffle or even the premonition of a sniffle was assaulted by capsule upon capsule of increasingly potent versions of vitamin C. With a little effort you could consume the vitamin C equivalent of the entire citrus crop of Spain in a matter of days. Could anything withstand such a megavitamin onslaught?

In short, the answer is yes. The common cold seemed singularly nonplussed at its supposed savaging at the hands of vitamin C. When vitamin C was finally subjected to a large-scale, controlled study in the San Francisco area, the results were disappointing for the colored-urine set. In terms of frequency, severity, or duration of colds, those who chewed vitamin C were no better off than those who eschewed vitamin C. Vitamin C is as good as any other placebo, which means not very good at all.

Moreover, the other placebos allow you to contemplate your urine with less suspicion and wonder than is the case with vitamin C. What should have been a terminal kick in the groin to the vitamin C plague rarely reached the back pages of the newspapers. It's the old story that dog bites man is not newsworthy. When vitamin C was "the cure for the common cold," the newspapers did not have large enough front pages.

Promises, particularly from Nobel laureates, are always big news, no matter how irrational they are. In fact, the addition of an element of irrationality, particularly when it is of an exceedingly optimistic or pessimistic variety, makes their pronouncements even more newsworthy. When a vitaholic is confronted with the hard facts about vitamin C, his or her typical retort is that "it seems to work for me." Large enough doses of vitamins obviously have a marked strengthening effect on credulity. Vitamin C sales are still quite brisk.

The "it works for me" illogic is hard to uproot. It is strengthened by the undeniable fact that there are considerable differences in the way individuals respond to almost any treatment. An important part of modern medicine is discovering the mechanisms for these individual differences and capitalizing on them to design optimal therapies. This research has already yielded some interesting and valuable points of general applicability. One is that the individual differences almost exclusively lie along a dimension of potency of effects. For example, certain doses of drugs may be virtually ineffective in some people and almost lethal in other people who are apparently no different.

Individual differences can enhance or inhibit the actions of almost any therapeutic agent. The critical point here is that there must be some significant action of the substance in the first place. Vitamin C has been shown to be absolutely ineffective in combating colds at any dose in anyone under controlled conditions. The fact that people think vitamin C is effective for them is likely to reflect the nature of their own uncontrolled self-experimentation. Either that or the idiosyncratic person is fundamentally different from the rest of humanity. Until the former possibility is explored, assuming that the latter is the case is silly and counterproductive. Of course we all value our own uniqueness, but we are all subject to the same law of gravity.

To overstate and misinterpret individual differences in response to medical treatment is to advocate a fundamental anarchy. If you do not wish there to be any order in the universe, you are unlikely to perceive any. Even if you do perceive order, you are likely to reject that which you do see. On the other hand, we have abundant evidence of all sorts of order at all levels of life. Whether you find this order philosophically comforting or repugnant is irrelevant. The basic facts are undeniable.

To assume a fundamental anarchy in health treatments is to don the intellectual blinders that characterize the health food movement. It is not a movement of optimism or of the future. It is fighting a rearguard action against reality. Even megalentils can't keep reality at bay for long. This movement is a new obscurantism, a frightened denial that seeks to substitute dogma and ignorance for logic and inquiry. Along the way, a lot of people are getting cheated and hurt.

Much of the harm caused by this obscurantism is that it buries a great deal that is important and exciting. Some real breakthroughs are on the horizon, but they are difficult to distinguish in an atmosphere so polluted with quackery. For example, there are now good data showing that many types of cancer have very different distributions in different countries. That these are not simply racial or ethnic differences is indicated by migration studies. Migrants who move from A to B generally end up showing cancer statistics like those of the people who had lived in area B all along. This raises the exciting possibility that situational factors such as diet are a major determinant of cancer. The same logic likely applies to many other diseases as well.

The nuts-and-raisins brigade have leaped upon epidemiological data such as these and ridden off in all directions at once. Typical of the red herrings that what their enthusiastic ignorance has led to is the supposed inhibiting effect that low body weight has on cancer. They support this claim by data from certain African groups who are subject to almost constant semistarvation. These groups have a very low incidence of cancer. This finding by itself precipitated a whole new wave of fasting and purging. Nothing is more evocative and frightening than the word *cancer*.

In their haste to get there quickly, the starvation advocates neglected to note several important points about the data that they were using. The main one is that, largely because of their chronic malnutrition, the life expectancy of the African people whom they were trying to emulate is extremely low. The reason they have relatively little cancer is that very few of them survive long enough for cancer to afflict them. If you looked at children who died before the age of ten, the incidence of cancer would be much lower still. Would you like to maintain that the miserable conditions of hygiene and poor health care that caused the high attrition rate in childhood be recommended to the rest of us as a cancer preventative?

It turns out that there is an astonishing array of agents that are natural carcinogens (cancer promoters) and anticarcinogens. Nearly every food that we eat contains these substances. New ones are being discovered every day. One titillating feature that many of the carcinogens have in common is that they liberate oxygen radicals. How this can lead to cancer need not sidetrack us here, but it is widely believed that it can. A few of these substances are in almost any damaged vegetable, burned or browned food, rhubarb, many fats and oils, and alfalfa sprouts. Consequently, it might seem prudent to avoid any foods that liberate oxygen radicals.

Conversely, a number of substances have the property of trapping or immobilizing oxygen radicals. This would, of course, be expected to exert an anticarcinogenic effect. A few of these natural anticarcinogens are carrots, cabbage, selenium, as well as the vitamins A, E, and C! Consequently, it might seem prudent to maximize your intake of these substances.

Although these data are fairly well established, just how one can translate them into action in terms of dietary changes is not at all clear. Of course, what the health food fraternity wants is action now. They are not at all interested in academic equivocating. Their health is on the line. Please note that in the above paragraphs where the suggestion was raised of a possibility of changing dietary practices, it was prefaced with an emphasized *might*.

There are many good reasons why these findings are only titillating and, for the moment at least, cannot be translated into viable action, no matter how urgent the need might be. One is the simple reason that we may well already have optimal levels of some of these anticarcinogenic substances. If this were the case, then increasing their levels might even reduce their effectiveness. Further, in the case of substances like selenium, even small doses are very toxic. It is often the case in nutrition that more does not necessarily mean better.

Maximizing antioxidants and minimizing oxidants in the diet is impossible to do on any rational grounds. The reason is that these substances almost invariably occur in complex mixtures of dozens, scores, or hundreds of other ingredients. This means that you can never just change your intake of these two classes of target compounds. When you change your diet substantially, you inevitably change the balance among hundreds of substances. How this unavoidable imbalance would affect the activity of oxidants and antioxidants cannot, at the moment, even be guessed at.

The basic problem is that we do not even really know much

about how the suspected oxidants and antioxidants act in isolation. To even hazard a guess about how they might interact in the complex mixtures in which they occur in the human body is premature. To experiment on yourself on the basis of such preliminary findings is not just premature, it could be very dangerous.

Statistically speaking, the chances of randomly disrupting any natural function are vastly greater than the chances of enhancing that function. At the moment, any of our activities with respect to modifying the ratio of oxidants to antioxidants are only crude guesswork at best. This means that they have a much greater likelihood of being harmful than helpful. In other words, you are more likely to increase your chances of getting cancer than to decrease them. The cost of making mistakes when you are playing with cancer can be total. This is no game for amateur experimentation, no matter how noble one's intentions are. Unfortunately, this is just what the health food movement is—amateur nutrition.

One of the hallmarks in this movement is a naive faith in the benevolence of natural processes. The buzzword *natural* has been worked to death. This delusional system has an unshakable belief that natural is good and not natural is bad. It is all part of a rejection of consumerism and the twentieth century as well. Nature is by no means the passive, benevolent entity these people believe it to be. The toughness and occasional downright nastiness of nature is summarized in the old saw "Nice guys finish last."

In order to protect themselves, all of the nuts, raisins, and other things in nature's garden had to develop defense mechanisms. Since plants cannot run and hide, they had very few options to protect themselves against predation from animals, other plants, and disease. Only plants that could regularly run this gamut of natural selection survived to be plucked and processed for your local health food store. All of the plant "nice guys" were evolutionary dead ends.

The main way plants have of protecting themselves is to develop their own toxins and pesticides. These chemical defense mechanisms vary enormously in potency. Some of them are among the most toxic and carcinogenic known. In many respects, synthetic toxins and carcinogens are often rather pale imitations of their natural cousins. After all, nature has been working at making these nasty substances much longer than we have.

Relatively few plants are toxic for all species, but nearly all are toxic for some species. Humans and all other species quickly learn to avoid frankly poisonous foods. This is one of the fastest and most universal forms of learning. This form of learning is made easy by the fact that the unpleasant consequences of poisoning always follow closely after eating the poison food. Quite simply, you know what made you ill.

On the other hand, carcinogenesis is an extraordinarily complex process that depends upon interactions among a large number of ill-understood variables. This means that the development of the nasty consequences of eating something carcinogenic is both slow and uncertain. You are not likely to know what might have given you cancer. It is hard to imagine any species learning to avoid something whose unpleasant consequences are so remote and variable.

The net result of these very poor conditions for learning is that neither humans nor any other species have developed a protective mechanism for avoiding carcinogenic foods. Until the multitude of natural carcinogens is identified, we are at the mercy of chance. The bright side of this picture is that there is substantial progress being made in this area, and it is being made not because of, but in spite of the health food faddists. They have done nothing positive to contribute to this new field of research. To the contrary, their gospel of doctrinaire obscurantism is only an impediment to real developments in this most important area. Faith and earnest rhetoric are no substitutes for evidence. Unfortunately, faith and rhetoric are all the health food movement has to offer.

The natural pesticides and carcinogens are present in virtually all foods and often at surprisingly high concentrations. The net result of this unavoidable soup of natural pesticides is that we eat a dietary intake of several grams of it per day. This is probably at least ten thousand times greater than our dietary intake of synthetic pesticides and carcinogens. These figures suggest that the obsessional attitude that prevails in the health food community about chemical fertilizers and pesticides may be a little off base.

The natural-health movement has sought to make *chemical* a dirty word. This is an absurd and counterproductive form of ignorance. It makes about as much sense as casting stones at gravity. That cherished prototype of the natural food, the apple, contains over two hundred chemicals in its flavor alone! Those who advocate "organic" farming would have us believe that a potato can tell whether the nitrogen it thrives on comes from horse manure or a bag of chemical fertilizer. The very notion of this sort of discrimination is absurd. Nitrogen is nitrogen, no matter how it is packaged. The suspicion of chemical fertilizers might be justified if the additional ingredients in the package were harmful. However, chemical fertilizers are really squeaky clean in this respect. Horse manure is far more likely to have all sorts of unpleasant contaminants than is most bagged fertilizer.

The fact that there have been some poor, perhaps even dangerous, chemical fertilizers does not detract from their overall value. The ineffective and dangerous kinks in fertilizers were worked out long ago. These products are, to a large extent, responsible for the miracles of modern agriculture. There is also a belief that organically grown vegetables are superior in flavor to the farm-factory variety. This may be so in certain countries such as the United States, but it is not a necessary truth. With many of the products of mass farming, the lack of flavor reflects a number of factors, of which fertilizer is only one. Mass-produced tomatoes, for example, may be inferior in taste because they were developed for many other properties besides flavor. Productivity, good color, resistance to disease, and an ability to withstand abusive handling are not necessarily compatible with the best flavor.

To attribute the flavor deficiency of mass-produced fruits and vegetables to the use of chemical fertilizers is not justified. The vacancy of this prejudice is shown by the fact that the fruits and vegetables of France, which are generally superior in flavor to those of the English-speaking countries, are all fertilized extensively from the bag. The suggestion to a French farmer that the equine fertilizer product is superior to the bagged variety is greeted with howls of derision.

The superior flavor of organically grown products is a fiction. It is a simple prejudice supported by no data at all. The same applies to allegations about the supposedly superior nutritional value of these products. There has never been a shred of evidence that organically grown food is any more nutritious than any other food.

Because of their doctrinaire avoidance of any plant sprays, organic farmers may well provide products that are not just more expensive and no more flavorful or nutritious than the other stuff, they may well be more dangerous too. One of the consistent findings of recent research is that the natural carcinogens and pesticides produced by plants are greatly increased by any damage to the plant. Since organically grown plants are not sprayed, they are inevitably more susceptible to being damaged by insects and plant diseases. This means that they are much more likely to be high in natural carcinogens and natural pesticides.

This is hardly the way to go about producing health food. Like all of the other claims for health foods, the claims for their lack of toxicity as compared with the supermarket products are not supported by any evidence. The evidence points in the other direction. Once again, these people ask us to believe them and ignore any dissonant information.

However much faith and goodwill you have, there is always a final reckoning. Organically grown foods must inevitably come to grips with the fundamental issue of whether they are in fact, as opposed to in claim, better. The foregoing analysis suggests that organically grown foods are no more nutritious or flavorful and are very likely more dangerous than their supermarket equivalents. Considering the fact that they are uniformly more expensive than the mainstream competition, they are a pretty awful product. The fact that they still sell fairly well is testimony to the deterioration in nutritional rationality that the health food industry has engendered.

In the race to be more organic than thou, large numbers of people have taken to macrobiotic diets. Many of these converts have found this diet while on the rebound from nasty experiences with drugs. Macrobiotics is based on Buddhist principles originally articulated by George Ohsawa. It is more than a diet, it is a whole philosophy of life. According to this view, disease is an expression of an imbalance between the two basic and essentially opposite principles, yin and yang.

Perhaps the most compelling feature of this diet is that, after subscribing to it, you do not have to think at all. The components of the diet, their nutritional value, how much you eat, when you eat, how you eat, and why you eat are all decided for you. The diet goes through ten stages of increasing rigor. In the last stage you eat nothing other than brown rice, each mouthful of which is chewed fifty times. This feast is to be washed down with no more than eight ounces of fluid per day. This is the perfect balance of yin and yang. At this stage they claim that you will be both disease-free and fully enlightened.

The popularity of this diet attests to the solid authoritarian streak that maintains so much of this nonsense. Notions like yin and yang may be acceptable in certain philosophical circles, but their application to nutrition is ridiculous. There is not even the faintest notion about what makes anything either yin or yang, let alone how you can work out this core principle for yourself. Since there is no official yin-yang center, I assume that there is someone who passes judgments on all foods. Do they just guess, or are they perhaps so enlightened that the judgments come to them spontaneously? Whatever the secret is, they are not letting it out. Your job is to sit there and listen. If any thinking is needed, they will take care of it.

This sort of diet is more than just mindless stupidity, it can be very dangerous. Brown rice is great stuff, but it is not, by itself, an adequate diet. Nor is this inadequacy compensated for by meditation. No matter how enlightened and ethereal you are, you still have minimal nutritional requirements. These minimal requirements are not met by a brown rice diet. The obsessional pursuit of enlightenment through brown rice has cost a number of people their lives. Others have escaped with kwashiorkor, a severe protein-deficiency disease usually found only in the poorest countries of the Third World. A 100 percent hamburger-and-soft-drink diet would be far healthier. It would likely be less stunting to your intellect as well.

With so much flagrant craziness in nutrition, it is little wonder that an increasing number of people are just turning away from it all in disgust. The idea of self-inflicted idiocy in the pursuit of mindless definitions of health and wisdom is repugnant to many thinking people. Through the process of aging, many of us will become stupid enough in the long run anyhow. To jump the gun and get on the senility bandwagon early is not particularly attractive.

This new wave of nutritional nihilism is the inevitable response to the rise in wide-eyed credulity I have just been describing. The new nihilism is unfortunate, because there are some genuine health benefits to be obtained by many people from adopting sound nutritional practices. The fact that these real nutritional benefits travel in close company with such quackery debases the whole subject matter.

The largest group in the entire health food movement is made up of vegetarians and the variations on that theme. This group has suffered from their associations with the organic, macrobiotic, and megavitamin messiahs. Vegetarianism also suffers from a host of religious associations that many would rather forget. These religious associations have given vegetarianism a rather haphazard, patchwork philosophical framework that makes many people uncomfortable.

Questions of rationale and philosophy aside, the real issue is, does vegetarianism have any real health benefits to offer? Here the answer is a qualified yes. The qualification results from the fact that although being vegetarian may be good for you, it is not really clear whether these benefits are due to eating less meat or to eating more good things that are not meat. This is not a trivial issue, since it means that an ill-advised vegetarian could eat a diet that is unhealthy. Conversely, a well-advised carnivore could eat a very healthy diet. It is not so much what you exclude as what you include.

The great majority of responsible nutritionists agree on the fact that most people eat too much protein, too many saturated fats, and too little complex carbohydrates and fibers. One way to solve this imbalance is to substitute grains, bread, pasta, and vegetables for meat. This is not the only way, it is merely a more obvious one. This substitution can be either total or partial and it can include or exclude fish and poultry. The precise mixture is not very important, but the effects of this sort of change may be quite valuable.

A vegetarian diet frequently produces large reductions in serum cholesterol and greatly improves the way other fats are handled. It can also improve glucose tolerance in diabetics and marginal diabetics. It also may reduce high blood pressure. All these effects are generally desirable and they occur in many people who change to vegetarian and semivegetarian diets. None of these is invariable, but the overall effect is far more than just another placebo effect. A vegetarian diet is not the road to enlightenment or to eternal life. Just the same it may be pretty good stuff.

Alas, as is the case with nearly everything that comes into even remote contact with issues of weight loss and nutrition, vegetarianism has its own quack wing. Zealous converts have made wild and ridiculous claims for the benefits to be gained from lentilism. The list of hyperboles should be familiar by now. A vegetarian diet will improve your sex life (this is always a big drawing card), bring about weight loss, destroy cellulite, stop hair loss, improve your complexion, oh and make you live for ever or nearly. This nonsense is based on no real information, only ignorance, enthusiasm, and credulity. As with all militant nonsense, it does a disservice to the real benefits that can be gained from this diet.

What is important about the health benefits of a vegetarian diet is that they occur quite independently of any changes in weight. Some people do lose weight on a vegetarian diet, but it is usually a transient loss. The health benefits to be reaped from this sort of diet do not require weight loss. It's just as well, since, as we already know, weight loss is a rare and elusive beast. Further, in many cases, even if weight loss is achieved, it is doubtful that it will be of any real health benefit.

This "new nutrition" advocated by the health food industry is not new at all. It is merely a repackaging of the same old amalgam of ignorance and greed that flourishes wherever there is human woe to be exploited. Neither the cause of nor the cure for any significant disease even approaches the childlike simplicity the health food movement would have us believe. They have got it all wrong in almost every significant respect. The result of their militant obscurantism is that they have thoroughly muddied the water. The relationship between nutrition, health, and disease is an important and exciting area. Progress in this area is being made in spite of, not because of, the health food movement.

Fat and Healthy

The antifat crusaders have been successful in stamping in the false belief that fat is synonymous with both ugliness and unhealthiness. The idea that fat is ugly is a value judgment. Subjective evaluations are merely statements of feeling. They may be silly or even harmful, but they cannot be wrong. This is why they are often so resistant to change. On the other hand, the idea that fat is unhealthy purports to be a statement of fact. Since it is an incorrect statement, it should be somewhat easier to overturn. Nevertheless, removing the stigma from fat and placing it in its proper perspective will be a long and arduous task.

The idea that fat people are definitionally unhealthy is firmly embedded in nearly every aspect of our culture. Fatness is portrayed as a disease latent in all of us. The slightest lapse in dietary vigilance may precipitate it. Once unleashed, gluttony and sloth produce a harvest of demon fat that is difficult to control. The price we pay for loss of control is a certain deterioration of health. Nearly everyone believes that fat people lead brief and blighted existences. This is the gospel of the antifat crusaders and it has become a central element in our social value system. Fat people are believed to be not only ugly but unhealthy and vice-ridden as well. Part of this gospel is that nearly everyone is too fat for his or her own good. This is in spite of an abundance of data indicating that the great majority of moderately fat people have nothing to worry about.

- Very few people are too fat.
- Fat people can be healthy.
- Fat people can be beautiful.

It is time the repugnant and destructive set of prejudices about fat was driven from the marketplace. Every aspect of this prejudicial edifice is based on demonstrably false or misinterpreted information. It is little consolation that those who have contributed most to the antifat prejudices may have done so with good intentions. Ignorance and misinformation are harmful irrespective of intentions. The net result of this fanaticism is both ugly and unhealthy. Fat people cannot be frightened or shamed into losing weight. This approach has been tried for a long time.

- Fear and loathing of fat are unjustified.

All that the antifat hysteria has done is to produce a generation of harassed and frightened people. Those who are already fat are frightened for their lives and many of those who are slim live in mortal fear of becoming fat. The fear of fat is making millions unhappy and unhealthy. Moreover, the size of this needlessly afflicted group is increasing. The population of the developed world is fatter than ever before and the slim people are more frightened than ever of becoming fat.

- People are becoming steadily fatter.
- The general increase in fatness is not an epidemic.

The worldwide trend toward increasing fatness is, to a large extent, responsible for the use of the label *epidemic*. This logic is wrong. There is no good reason to consider the general increase in fatness an epidemic. People are becoming taller, too, but nobody talks about a height epidemic. Nor is there any good reason to consider fatness a disease. The people of the Western world are both fatter and healthier than ever before.

- People are both fatter and healthier than ever before.
- Most people are frightened of their own bodies.

The medical profession and a giant fat-exploitation industry have failed miserably in their attempts to eradicate fatness. They have not only failed to eradicate it, they have failed to slow its rate of increase. There has never been an epidemic of any type that has been so completely unresponsive to such an enormous and sustained international effort. The great traditional killers tuberculosis, cancer, and heart disease have all responded to a broad-based medical attack. In developed countries tuberculosis is nearly eradicated and deaths from cancer and heart disease are steadily decreasing. In marked contrast, fatness has been considered to be a killer disease for at least thirty or forty years. In spite of an immense international campaign at both the clinical and the basic-research level, fatness is clearly on the increase. Either fatness is the most difficult major health problem of all time, or its potential to harm has been seriously overestimated.

Much of this book has tried to make the point that fatness is not usually a health problem. That is not to say that fatness is never a health problem, just that it is a genuine problem for only a small percentage of those who are worried about it.

- Most adults are worried about their weight.
- Few adults should be worried about their weight.

The singular failure of the antifat industry to do anything about fat other than frighten people about it suggests that fat may not really be the problem they portray it to be. The hysterical opposition to fat in any form is not justified. The antifat industry has thoroughly muddied the issue by confusing fat that is a health concern with fat that is simply fat and is nothing to be worried about. Fat is probably only a genuine health concern for groups that suffer from the following conditions:

- Massive obesity
- Diabetes
- Cardiovascular disease
- High cholesterol levels

There is clear evidence that being fat is unhealthy, even dangerous for these groups. If you fall into any of these groups, it is better not to be fat. However, there is no evidence at all that fatness *causes* any of the above problems. In particular, there is little evidence that fatness causes diabetes, cardiovascular disease, or high cholesterol levels. This important distinction is usually lost in the general outcry against fat. This, of course, means that even in the unlikely event that fatness were eradicated, it would have little or no effect on the incidence of these diseases. Eradicating fatness would certainly help such people, but it would do relatively little to reduce the occurrence of these diseases. Of course, this is all merely wishful thinking anyhow, since it is highly unlikely that fatness will ever be eliminated, or even substantially reduced. Influential groups such as the American Heart Association do the cause of public health a disservice by conveying the impression that weight loss is both desirable and possible for almost anyone. Instead, the reality is that weight loss is only occasionally desirable and very rarely possible for anyone.

- Most people would be no healthier if they lost weight.
- Weight loss is not possible for most people.

Those who could genuinely profit from losing weight (the massively obese, diabetics, and those with cardiovascular or cholesterol problems) are those for whom weight loss is generally most difficult. Although fat-endangered people cannot often lose weight, they can almost always show real health benefits from both exercise and sound dietary practice. In contrast to weight loss, the following will improve the health of almost anyone:

- Stopping smoking
- Reasonable and regular exercise
- Increased carbohydrate intake
- Decreased saturated fat intake

The almost exclusive preoccupation with fat as the culprit in all health problems is very unhealthy. It is doubly unfortunate since the hysteria has largely been generated by groups that profess the greatest concern with public health. To indiscriminately advocate weight loss when it is not generally attainable is stress-producing and unhealthy. It is just this sort of misguided prescription that has lead to a steady loss of public confidence in the medical profession. It is little wonder that in such a confused and frightened situation the health charlatans have thrived.

A generation of failed dieters is adequate testimony to the fact that adjuring people to lose weight is usually done in vain. It is further testimony to the fact that diets and exercise are not good ways to lose weight. The steady improvement in public health is straightforward testimony to the fact that the dangers of fatness are far overstated.

- Dieting is not a good way to lose weight.
- Exercise is not a good way to lose weight.

In contrast to the elusive goal of weight loss, sound life-style, exercise, and sensible dietary practices are easily within the reach of nearly everyone. The antifat messiahs have incorrectly labeled the general increase in fatness an epidemic. They have prescribed ineffective treatments for what is generally not a problem in the first place. The public has developed a morbid fear of eating because it firmly believes that overeating is the road to fatness and perdition. The evidence does not support this common fear. Most fat people do not overeat, and undereating (dieting) is not a generally effective way to lose weight.

The public paranoia about food has generated one of the biggest nutritional frauds of all time—the health food myth. Flagrantly unsound and dangerous nutritional practices are a genuine epidemic. The antifat messiahs both indirectly and directly lend support to an astonishing array of crazy, ineffective, and harmful dietary practices. In an atmosphere of such lunacy, it is little wonder that sound nutritional advice is frequently paid little heed. Failed and frightened dieters are prime candidates for unhealthy, desperate, treatments, such as smoking, drugs, starvation, and surgery. When these treatments also fail, thoroughly defeated dieters often abandon all nutritional caution and become junk-food fiends. At the same time, they are likely to abstain from all forms of exercise. All of this is clearly unhealthy and clearly avoidable if they were not so weight-obsessed. The purpose of this book is to destroy the obsession with weight. Health is only possible when we learn to live with and not against our bodies.

- Fatness is not generally a disease.

Instead of fatness being a new epidemic, we are probably merely witnessing a gradual shift to a new body-composition profile for most of our species. The reasons for this shift may take a long time to determine, but if it is a natural shift, the implications are straightforward. Such a natural shift would likely be nearly irresistible.

We have already stressed that this relatively laissez-faire attitude toward fat does not apply to diabetics and those with cardiovascular or cholesterol problems. Nor does it apply to the massively obese. Fortunately, only a tiny percentage of fat people are massively obese. The great majority of the fat population is just modestly overweight. Gross fatness may well indicate some underlying disease process, and this sort of fatness certainly is a health hazard. If half of your body weight is fat, the fat is likely to compromise breathing and place a major strain on nearly every physiological system. However, there is no indication of any sudden and large increase in massive obesity. Moderate fatness is on the increase, but the incidence of massive obesity remains quite constant. Nor has there been any real progress in the treatment of gross obesity. These genuinely unfortunate people get far more attention now than ever before, but there is little indication of any general improvement in their lot.

Even the last resort, gastric surgery, for morbid obesity is at best a faint hope. It is not yet clear whether such surgery really results in an overall improvement in the health status of the massively obese.

- Antifat surgery is both experimental and dangerous.
- Drugs are not effective in facilitating weight loss.

Continued efforts to find an effective treatment for fatness is justified by the existence of the massively obese, diabetics, and those who have either cardiovascular or cholesterol problems. If such a treatment is found, it is to be hoped that its use will be restricted to that small group for whom weight loss is a health imperative. To try to defeat human physiology for cosmetic purposes is likely to do more harm than good.

The antifat messiahs and the medical profession have incorrectly deduced from the ill health of the massively obese that any degree of fatness is dangerous and unhealthy. This is not logically correct, and more importantly, health data do not support their negative view. The main reason why fat people tend to be unhealthy is not their fat as such, but other factors, such as improper diet and exercise along with high blood pressure and high cholesterol levels. It is crucial to note, however, that there is no indication that either high blood pressure or high cholesterol levels is caused by fatness. The extent of the fat madness is indicated by the fact that fat people often smoke in an attempt to control their weight.

Fat has been incorrectly held to cause all sorts of health problems, whereas it is usually merely an exacerbating factor. Even then most people are unjustifiably frightened of their fat.

A very large percentage of those who are said to be too fat for their own good are 10 to 30 percent over some ideal weight. It is becoming increasingly clear that this level of fatness is more benign that the public has been led to believe. This is particularly true in women. Women clearly have the least to fear from fat, and yet are the most terrorized by it.

If you are fat today, you will probably be fat tomorrow. Just because fatness is usually a permanent state, it does not mean that most fat people cannot be healthy. There is no good reason why the vast majority of fat people have to lead either brief or blighted existences. It is a gratifying sign of change that some of the more enlightened physicians are finally giving fat people who come to them some really useful advice. They are telling them that although they probably can't help them to become thin, they may be able to help them be healthy.

For millennia *fat* and *healthy* were considered synonymous. For a scant generation, fatness and good health have been held to be mutually exclusive. The monumental failure to stop fat is gradually leading to a revival of the old lore. It is very difficult to do much about fat, but it is quite easy to improve the health of most fat people. Fat people no longer have to be the passive victims of a cruel fate. They can now become active agents and take charge of their own healthy future. This process can be divided into a number of fairly distinct stages.

First comes the stage of resistance. It is just possible that when an undesired amount of fat appears on you, it is a transient and reversible process. Alternatively, it may simply be the emergence of the real you. The only way to find out is to see how your fat responds to your efforts to shake it.

- Try a sensible diet as a personal experiment.
- Diets probably won't help, but they don't have to hurt either.

Any well-balanced diet that is low in energy content will bring about a state of negative energy balance. This will challenge your fat. If you stick to the diet for a while and lose little or no weight, your body may be trying to tell you something. Similarly, if you do lose some weight and then rapidly put it back on after stopping the diet, you may be getting the same message. Fat could be your destiny.

If a diet doesn't work, don't despair. You should not expect it to work in the first place.

- There are no secrets to losing weight.
- There are real ways to improve your health.

When your diet fails, remember that there are further courts of appeal. Try a different diet. Just make sure it is reasonably well balanced. Another diet may be sufficiently different in macronutrient composition to facilitate metabolic changes that will bring about weight loss. The name of the game in weight loss is negative energy balance.

- Real weight loss requires metabolic adjustments.
- What controls metabolism is not yet certain.

The goal of negative energy balance is usually defeated by metabolic reductions in response to diets. Just what triggers the metabolic compensation to diets is not yet clear, but there is always the hope that some new diet may succeed where the others have failed by virtue of avoiding the metabolic compensation. There may be a diet that for you will minimize the metabolic compensation that normally defeats attempts to lose weight. The whole issue of differences in metabolic responses to macronutrients and micronutrients of various diets is just beginning to be explored. You may be lucky and find a metabolic key that is just right for you. It is not likely, but it is possible. At any rate, if a diet is approached as an experiment with yourself and not as a measure of your moral worth, it can do little harm.

It is probably a good idea if you accompany dietary resistance with some exercise. The energy value of the exercise probably won't help much (see chapter 6), but exercise might just help turn that resistant metabolic key. If you don't really expect much in the way of weight loss in the first place, you will only be minimally disappointed.

It is now clear that minor weight adjustments of, say, ten or even twenty pounds are feasible for many people. They require no magic, just negative energy balance. It is equally clear that larger amounts of weight loss will only be achieved by a tiny minority (less than 3 percent) of those who try.

There are two, quite distinct steps that must be taken in order to lose weight permanently. First, you have to achieve a stage of negative energy balance, which will shed the excess fat. Then you must revert to a state of neutral energy balance, which will permanently prevent the reaccumulation of fat. Because fat has such a high energy value, shedding fat (as opposed to water) is a slow, laborious process.

- Starvation diets are dangerous and counterproductive.

Forget starvation, semistarvation, and other crazy, unbalanced diets. They are almost certain to make things more difficult in the long run. They may even be dangerous. There is an accumulating body of evidence that suggests that starvation diets and all of the variants on that theme merely act to train your metabolic compensation mechanisms so that successive attempts at losing weight are progressively more difficult.

If, at the end of a reasonable sequence of diets (say, 2,000 to 2,500 kcal), accompanied by some exercise, you can not maintain an acceptable weight you have probably lost the game. If maintaining your new weight requires the permanent adoption of semistarvation, your diet is not likely to be a long-term success. While it is just possible for some fanatics to survive this way, it is probably not a healthy way to live. This kind of dietary fanaticism may be justified in certain defined medical conditions (see chapter 2), but it is not a desirable aim for most of the population. This is perhaps just as well, since only a very tiny percentage of the population is capable of substantial long-term privation. It should be reiterated that for dieting to be successful in the long term, it must be a permanent way of life. The idea of the "quicky" diet is a cruel illusion for most people. Temporary diets only produce temporary results at best.

Failure at this stage, or at any other for that matter, does not mean that you are a failure as a person. It does, however, mean that you are probably destined to be a fat person.

- Some people are simply meant to be fat.
- Fat is not failure.

Being a failed dieter makes you a member of a very large club. To fail at dieting is the norm. To succeed at dieting is a rarity. In either case, failing or succeeding at dieting says nothing about your character or moral worth. It does, however, say something about your basic physiology.

The next stage is acceptance. This should not be confused with the dejected resignation that eventually overtakes most dieters. Acceptance is a positive realization that you are fat and are probably always going to be fat. Your fat is an expression of your fundamental physiology. It is not the symptom of any vice or personal deficiency. Acceptance of fat means that you are going to live a life with your fat, not against it.

Living with fat does not mean an abandonment of aesthetic standards or a rejection of your own sexuality. It means not capitulating to what you have been told all along.

- Fatness and thinness are neither virtues nor vices.

Thin people are neither superior nor inferior to fat people. They are merely different. Developing your own sense of beauty and sexuality will take time and the support of other people. Thin people certainly do not stand alone. Why should fat people? Here is where various fat-consciousness groups may be of value. It is gratifying that there is now a radio program in New York that is specifically targeted at fat women. There are several new books that are addressing the same problem. Things are changing, but it is a slow and sometimes painful process. Accepting your fat will not be easy. Old prejudices die hard. It is, however, the only way out of the fat wilderness.

Accepting your fat as a normal part of you, rather than as an alien pathology that afflicts you, means that you can start to think positively about your health. There are lots of things everyone can do to improve his or her health. Whether you are fat, thin, or in between, there are affirmative steps you can take.

These steps include stopping smoking as a very first and essential measure. Another step is obvious, yet generally ignored: Regular medical examinations are invaluable in providing early warning of the development of any danger signs. In addition, a number of valuable nutritional truths are emerging. Eating a sensible diet is now easier than ever before. Amid all the nutritional quackery there is still a lot of sound and useful information that can benefit almost anyone. High-carbohydrate, low-animal-fat diets, perhaps coupled with regular eating of fish, are beginning to look increasingly good. Certainly, hundreds of millions of residents of the Orient and the Mediterranean countries would testify that such diets can also be aesthetically gratifying. Couple this with a good exercise program and you have a pretty good package. It's healthy and enjoyable. This approach stands in stark contrast to the privation, purge, and penance advocated by the health and weight-loss merchants who currently dominate the marketplace. This sort of program could even help you to lose a little weight, but as we have maintained before, the weight itself is generally not very important. If these nutritional and life-style patterns are superimposed on a genuine acceptance of who and what you are, you will finally have achieved freedom from fat.